STILLMAN DIET FOR WEIGHT LOSS

The All-in-One Guide for Eliminating Diabetes, Shedding Fat with Low Carb, High Protein Recipes

Audrey McAllister, MD

Requests for permission to use or reproduce any part of this publication should be addressed to the publisher in writing. The publisher reserves the right to grant or deny permission at their discretion, taking into consideration factors such as the intended use, nature of the excerpt, and potential impact on the original work.

Unauthorized reproduction or distribution of copyrighted material is a violation of intellectual property rights and may result in legal consequences. Individuals or entities found to be in breach of copyright law may be subject to legal action, including but not limited to injunctions, damages, and legal fees.

It is the responsibility of all users of this publication to familiarize themselves with and abide by copyright laws and regulations. By accessing or using any part of this work, individuals agree to comply with the terms and conditions set forth by the publisher regarding copyright protection and usage rights.

Table of Contents

INTRODUCTION

In the vast landscape of dietary philosophies and weight loss Directionologies, the Stillman Diet stands as a beacon of innovation and possibility. Conceived by Dr. Irwin Maxwell Stillman in the 1960s, this transformative approach to nutrition has left an indelible mark on the realm of health and wellness. As we embark on an exploration of the Stillman Diet, we are not merely delving into a regimen of meal plans and food restrictions but stepping into a legacy of discovery, perseverance, and enduring impact.

At its core, the Stillman Diet is distinguished by its simplicity and focus on high-protein, low-carbohydrate consumption. Dr. Stillman recognized the profound influence of dietary macronutrients on metabolic processes and sought to harness this understanding to facilitate rapid weight loss and optimize overall health. Through a strategic combination of lean proteins and minimal carbohydrates, the Stillman Diet offers a pathway to recalibrate the body's metabolic machinery, igniting fat-burning mechanisms and promoting sustainable weight management.

In this comprehensive guide, we embark on a journey to uncover the principles, mechanisms, and potential benefits of the Stillman Diet. From its historical roots to its contemporary relevance, we delve into the evolution of this dietary approach and its enduring legacy in the field of nutrition science. Drawing upon scientific research, anecdotal evidence, and expert insights, we illuminate the intricacies of the Stillman Diet, empowering readers to make informed decisions and embark on their own transformative journeys.

Throughout our exploration, we will navigate the intricacies of protein metabolism, delve into the physiological responses elicited by low-carbohydrate intake, and examine the practical considerations of implementing the Stillman Diet in everyday life. We will also explore the broader implications of dietary interventions on metabolic health, exploring the potential synergies between nutrition, exercise, and lifestyle modifications in achieving optimal outcomes.

But beyond the scientific discourse lies a rich tapestry of human experience—a testament to the profound impact of the Stillman Diet on the lives of individuals around the world. Through firsthand accounts, success stories, and personal testimonies, we will glimpse the transformative power of this dietary approach, witnessing the triumphs, challenges, and moments of inspiration that have shaped the journeys of those who have embraced the Stillman Diet.

As we embark on this exploration of the Stillman Diet, we invite readers to approach with curiosity, open-mindedness, and a spirit of discovery. Whether you are seeking to shed excess weight, improve metabolic health, or simply deepen your understanding of nutrition and wellness, the insights gleaned from our exploration of the Stillman Diet promise to inform, inspire, and empower you on your quest for optimal health and vitality. So, let us embark together on this journey of exploration and enlightenment, as we unlock the secrets of the Stillman Diet and discover the transformative potential that lies within.

SECTION 1: DEMYSTIFYING THE STILLMAN DIET

The Stillman Diet, conceived by Dr. Irwin Maxwell Stillman during the 1960s, stands as a precursor to the contemporary low-carbohydrate diet movement and exerted a profound influence on subsequent dietary programs such as the Atkins Diet. Distinguished by its innovative fusion of low carbohydrate and high protein principles, this dietary regimen has garnered attention for its unique approach to weight management.

Central to the Stillman Diet is the emphasis on prioritizing protein-rich foods within daily dietary intake. Lean sources of protein, including poultry, seafood, eggs, and dairy, are commonly recommended staples. The diet imposes strict limitations on carbohydrate consumption, particularly targeting sugars, wheat, and starchy foods, with the aim of inducing ketosis—a metabolic state wherein the body predominantly utilizes stored fat for energy due to a scarcity of carbohydrates.

While the diet's carbohydrate restrictions are well-defined, guidelines regarding saturated fat consumption may vary. Notably, the Stillman Diet diverges from conventional calorie-counting approaches, instead placing greater emphasis on the quality and composition of food choices. The thermogenic effects associated with digesting protein are highlighted, suggesting that protein-rich selections may promote satiety and calorie expenditure, thereby facilitating weight management.

In addition to dietary recommendations, the Stillman Diet underscores the importance of adequate hydration by advocating for sufficient water intake.

Beyond mere hydration, adequate water consumption is believed to support waste elimination and overall metabolic function.

Despite the potential efficacy of restrictive diets like the Stillman Diet in achieving short-term weight loss goals, careful consideration must be given to their long-term implications and potential health risks. Prioritizing nutritional adequacy and minimizing adverse effects necessitates consultation with healthcare professionals before embarking on significant dietary changes.

In summary, while the Stillman Diet presents a structured approach to weight management with its focus on protein-rich foods and carbohydrate restriction, individuals are advised to approach it judiciously and seek personalized guidance to ensure optimal health outcomes in the long term.

What does the Stillman Diet entail?

Renowned for its core principles of advocating low-carbohydrate and high-protein consumption, the Stillman Diet emerged in the 1960s under the guidance of Dr. Irwin Maxwell Stillman. Central to its philosophy is the concept of curtailing carbohydrate intake while elevating protein intake. Serving as a precursor to subsequent low-carbohydrate dietary trends, the Stillman Diet remains a seminal influence in shaping modern dietary approaches.

A cornerstone of the Stillman Diet lies in the promotion of protein-rich foods, including eggs, dairy products, lean meats, fish, and poultry. These sources of protein are accorded special significance due to their satiating effect and thermogenic properties, whereby the body expends more energy digesting protein compared to other macronutrients.

Central to the Stillman Diet is a rigorous restriction on carbohydrates, particularly those derived from sugars, wheat, and starchy foods. By limiting carbohydrate intake, the diet aims to induce a metabolic state known as ketosis, wherein the body utilizes stored fat for energy instead of relying on carbohydrates. Proponents of this metabolic shift suggest that it may enhance fat burning and facilitate weight loss.

Despite its emphasis on food quality, the Stillman Diet typically does not advocate for stringent calorie tracking. While guidelines on fat consumption are not explicitly defined, recommendations may lean towards promoting unsaturated fats while limiting saturated fat intake.

As with any dietary regimen, the Stillman Diet presents both advantages and drawbacks. While some individuals may experience rapid weight loss, sustaining such a restrictive eating pattern over the long term can prove challenging. Moreover, considerations regarding potential nutrient deficiencies and overall health implications must be taken into account.

Given the complexities and potential risks associated with the Stillman Diet, it is prudent for individuals considering its adoption or similar dietary approaches to seek guidance from healthcare professionals. Consulting with a doctor can provide personalized insight into the suitability of such dietary modifications and help mitigate potential health risks.

In essence, while the Stillman Diet offers a structured approach to weight management, it is essential to approach it with caution and mindfulness towards individual health needs and long-term sustainability. By making informed decisions and seeking professional guidance, individuals can navigate dietary choices that align with their overall health and wellness goals.

The progression and development of the Stillman Diet over time.

An essential milestone in the annals of weight management strategies and nutritional Directionologies emerges with the advent of the Stillman Diet, credited to the pioneering efforts of Dr. Irwin Maxwell Stillman in the 1960s. Dr. Stillman, a renowned physician and obesity researcher, introduced this dietary regimen as a precursor to the low-carbohydrate, high-protein approaches that gained prominence in subsequent decades. At the time of its inception, the landscape of obesity research was undergoing significant evolution, prompting a quest for novel strategies in combating excess weight and promoting healthier lifestyles.

The distinctive feature of the Stillman Diet upon its introduction was its unprecedented emphasis on protein-rich meals. Dr. Stillman advocated for a dietary plan that prioritized lean protein sources such as chicken, fish, eggs, and dairy, while advocating for reduced carbohydrate intake. This departure from conventional nutritional wisdom, which traditionally advocated for a more balanced distribution of macronutrients, marked a paradigm shift in dietary recommendations for weight management.

The influence of the Stillman Diet reverberated through subsequent dietary trends, most notably with the rise of the Atkins Diet in the 1970s, which mirrored many of its fundamental principles and experienced a comparable surge in popularity. Although the Stillman Diet may not have sustained its initial level of acclaim over time, its contribution to our understanding of the interplay between macronutrient composition, metabolic function, and weight control cannot be understated.

As with many dietary fads, the Stillman Diet has undergone evolution and adaptation over the years, influenced by shifting trends and emerging scientific insights into nutrition and metabolism. While its prominence may have waned amidst the influx of new weight reduction Directionologies, the legacy of the Stillman Diet endures, leaving an indelible imprint on the realm of contemporary dietary practices.

Indeed, the Stillman Diet occupies a significant chapter in the chronicles of weight management programs, serving as a testament to the perpetual quest for effective and sustainable approaches to achieving optimal health and wellness. Its enduring impact is evidenced by the enduring interest in low-carbohydrate dietary patterns and the recognition of macronutrient composition as a crucial determinant in shaping dietary guidelines and recommendations.

In the ever-evolving landscape of nutritional science and weight management strategies, the Stillman Diet remains a pivotal milestone, embodying the spirit of innovation and inquiry that continues to drive progress in the field of public health and wellness. While newer Directionologies may emerge and prevailing paradigms may shift, the foundational contributions of the Stillman Diet endure as a cornerstone of modern nutrition and weight management practices.

SECTION 2: PRINCIPLES OF THE STILLMAN DIET

When it comes to achieving weight loss and managing dietary habits, the Stillman Diet abides by a set of core principles elucidated by Dr. Irwin Maxwell Stillman. These principles lay down specific guidelines for macronutrient consumption and meal selection, aiming to facilitate effective weight management.

Central to the Stillman Diet is the notion of prioritizing protein intake. Advocates of this dietary approach encourage individuals to incorporate ample amounts of protein-rich foods into their meals, including eggs, dairy products, lean meats, fish, and poultry. This emphasis stems from the understanding that protein possesses a thermogenic effect, whereby the body expends more energy during the digestion of protein compared to other macronutrients.

Furthermore, the Stillman Diet underscores the importance of reducing carbohydrate intake, particularly those derived from grains, sugars, and starchy foods. By limiting carbohydrates, the diet aims to induce a metabolic state known as ketosis, wherein the body utilizes stored fat for energy instead of relying on carbohydrates.

While the Stillman Diet does impose restrictions on fats, particularly certain types, its primary focus remains on controlling calorie intake for the purpose of weight reduction. The diet promotes the consumption of foods rich in lean protein while discouraging or restricting the intake of carbohydrate-heavy foods. Additionally, it allows for the inclusion of low-carbohydrate vegetables to achieve a more balanced nutritional profile.

Hydration is also emphasized within the Stillman Diet, with recommendations for individuals to drink ample amounts of water. This practice is believed to promote satiety, support the body's natural detoxification processes, and contribute to overall health and well-being.

Unlike some weight loss programs that emphasize meticulous calorie counting, the Stillman Diet places greater emphasis on the overall composition of the diet, operating under the assumption that a low-carbohydrate, high-protein approach inherently results in calorie restriction.

While often touted as an intensive weight loss plan, the effectiveness of the Stillman Diet may be limited over the long term. Concerns exist regarding the sustainability of weight loss achieved through this Direction and the potential for nutritional deficiencies. Despite its ability to yield rapid weight loss in the short term, individuals considering the Stillman Diet are urged to exercise caution and seek medical guidance before implementing significant changes to their eating habits.

In summary, the Stillman Diet advocates for a low-fat, high-protein approach with a focus on carbohydrate limitation. While appealing to those seeking quick results, it prioritizes food selection and composition over meticulous calorie tracking. Individuals contemplating embarking on the Stillman Diet should approach it cautiously, consulting with healthcare professionals to ensure its appropriateness for their individual needs and goals.

Advantages and Obstacles

The Stillman Diet, centered on the restriction of carbohydrates and the promotion of high protein intake, presents several potential benefits that individuals may find appealing. One notable advantage is the prospect of rapid weight loss, particularly during the initial phases of the diet. By focusing on protein-rich foods, individuals may experience enhanced satiety, making it easier to regulate calorie intake and potentially facilitate weight reduction. Additionally, proponents of the diet suggest that inducing ketosis, wherein the body utilizes its fat stores for energy, can accelerate fat burning and promote weight loss.

Moreover, the structured nature of the Stillman Diet, with its specific guidelines and recommendations, may offer a sense of reassurance for those who prefer a regimented approach to meal planning. Furthermore, proponents of the diet contend that it may assist individuals in overcoming cravings for refined carbohydrates and other unhealthy eating habits, thus improving adherence to the diet and overall health.

However, despite the potential advantages associated with the Stillman Diet, it is essential to consider the potential drawbacks and risks. One significant concern is the long-term sustainability of the diet. Given its emphasis on restricting certain food groups, such as fruits, vegetables, and whole grains, there is a risk of nutritional deficiencies, which can disrupt the body's natural balance and lead to inadequate intake of essential vitamins and minerals.

Furthermore, individuals with certain medical conditions, such as renal issues, may face exacerbated symptoms due to the high protein consumption advocated by the Stillman Diet. The strain on the kidneys from excessive protein intake can potentially worsen existing renal problems. Additionally, the restrictive nature of the diet may lead to boredom and dissatisfaction, as individuals may find themselves limited by the available food options and the potential for repetition.

Moreover, adhering to a restrictive diet like the Stillman Diet may pose social challenges, as it can limit participation in social gatherings and shared meals. This aspect may contribute to feelings of isolation and difficulty maintaining social connections, which can impact overall well-being.

Furthermore, a notable concern is the lack of a structured plan for transitioning off the diet beyond the initial phase. Without clear guidance on how to maintain weight loss and adopt a more sustainable eating pattern, individuals may struggle to sustain their progress and may be at risk of regaining lost weight.

In light of these considerations, while the Stillman Diet may offer an organized approach to weight loss and the potential for rapid results, it is crucial to be aware of the associated risks, including nutritional deficiencies, negative health effects, long-term viability, and social ramifications. Consulting with a healthcare practitioner is essential to ensure that nutritional needs are met and potential hazards are mitigated when following any restrictive diet plan.

SECTION 3: MACRONUTRIENT RATIOS IN THE STILLMAN DIET

The Stillman Diet is characterized by specific macronutrient ratios that prioritize high protein intake, restrict carbohydrate consumption, and moderate fat intake. The fundamental principle underlying this dietary approach is to induce a state of ketosis, wherein the body predominantly utilizes stored fat for energy due to limited carbohydrate availability. Consequently, the macronutrient distribution in the Stillman Diet typically entails abundant protein, moderate fat, and minimal carbohydrates.

Central to the Stillman Diet is the emphasis on protein as a primary macronutrient source. This dietary protocol encourages the consumption of protein-rich foods such as eggs, dairy products, lean meats, fish, and poultry. The prominence of protein serves dual purposes: supporting muscle maintenance and leveraging the thermogenic effect associated with protein digestion, potentially enhancing overall calorie expenditure.

In addressing carbohydrates, the Stillman Diet adopts a strategy of restriction by minimizing intake from carbohydrate-containing foods like grains, sweets, and starchy vegetables. By limiting carbohydrate intake, the diet aims to deplete glycogen stores and induce ketosis, a metabolic state purported to facilitate increased fat oxidation and promote weight loss.

While the Stillman Diet does not impose as stringent restrictions on fat consumption as it does on carbohydrates and protein, it advocates for mindful selection of fats. Guidance is provided to prioritize healthy fats over saturated fats, with an emphasis on sources such as nuts, seeds, avocados, and olive oil. This approach aims to optimize the quality of fat intake while aligning with overall health goals.

In essence, the macronutrient composition of the Stillman Diet entails a balanced distribution of fats, carbohydrates, and protein, with a notable emphasis on protein and restriction of carbohydrates to induce metabolic changes favoring fat utilization. However, it is essential for individuals considering embarking on the Stillman Diet to consult with healthcare professionals before initiation. These dietary modifications have the potential to disrupt the body's natural nutritional balance and may require careful supervision to ensure adequate nutrient intake and overall well-being.

The significance of foods high in protein

The Stillman Diet, much like numerous other dietary approaches, places considerable emphasis on the consumption of protein-rich foods, recognizing their pivotal role in sustaining essential biological functions and promoting overall health. A plethora of reasons underscores the significance of integrating these nutrient-dense foods—comprising lean meats, poultry, fish, eggs, and dairy—into one's dietary regimen.

At the core of protein's importance lies its role as the fundamental building blocks of biological structures, encompassing skeletal muscle, connective tissue, enzymes, and hormones. A diet abundant in protein is indispensable for facilitating various physiological processes, spanning tissue repair, muscular development, and immune system function, thereby supporting optimal health and well-being.

One notable advantage of incorporating protein-rich meals is their ability to induce satiety, owing to their slower digestion rate compared to fats and carbohydrates. This satiating effect aids in hunger regulation and caloric restriction, which is particularly beneficial for individuals striving to achieve or maintain a healthy weight, emphasizing the crucial role of protein in effective weight management strategies.

Furthermore, protein-rich foods contribute to energy expenditure through their thermogenic properties, whereby the process of digesting protein consumes more energy compared to other macronutrients. This heightened metabolic effect translates to increased calorie expenditure, thereby potentially facilitating weight loss efforts and promoting favorable changes in body composition.

Beyond their protein content, these foods serve as valuable sources of essential vitamins and minerals, enhancing the overall nutrient density and nutritional quality of meals. By incorporating a diverse array of protein sources into one's diet, individuals can ensure comprehensive nutrient intake, thereby supporting optimal health and vitality.

In the context of dietary regimens such as the Stillman Diet, protein-rich foods assume a central role due to their multifaceted benefits, including their role as structural components of bodily tissues, their influence on satiety and energy expenditure, and their contribution to overall nutritional balance. Prioritizing muscle health and nutritional adequacy, a diet rich in protein from varied sources holds promise in fostering holistic well-being.

Given the individualized nature of dietary requirements and health goals, it is imperative for individuals to consult with healthcare professionals or nutrition experts to tailor dietary strategies according to their unique needs and objectives. Through personalized guidance and informed decision-making, individuals can optimize their dietary choices to attain a balanced macronutrient intake and promote long-term health and wellness.

SECTION 4: HYDRATION IN THE STILLMAN DIET

The Stillman Diet, akin to any well-rounded dietary regimen, underscores the critical importance of maintaining proper hydration levels. While the primary focus of the Stillman Diet revolves around the manipulation of macronutrient intake, specifically emphasizing low carbohydrate intake and increased protein consumption, the significance of adequate hydration remains paramount.

Water, an essential component of bodily function, assumes an even greater role when dietary modifications are implemented. Adequate hydration facilitates the breakdown of food, enhances nutrient absorption, and facilitates the elimination of waste products. Given the emphasis on protein consumption inherent in the Stillman Diet, sufficient water intake becomes indispensable to support processes such as protein metabolism, prevent dehydration, and promote optimal kidney function.

Moreover, water serves as a potent appetite suppressant, aiding in the perception of fullness and potentially mitigating the risk of overeating. The tendency to mistake thirst for hunger is a common pitfall that can lead to excessive calorie consumption. Therefore, maintaining proper hydration levels becomes instrumental in effectively managing food intake, thus facilitating weight loss objectives, which are central to the Stillman Diet's goals.

Particularly noteworthy is the necessity for enhanced hydration when adhering to the Stillman Diet, as the reduction in carbohydrate intake induces a state of ketosis. During ketosis, the body experiences increased water and electrolyte loss, necessitating a corresponding increase in fluid intake to maintain optimal hydration and electrolyte balance. Failure to adequately hydrate while in ketosis can lead to adverse effects such as headaches, fatigue, and dehydration, underscoring the critical role of hydration management.

While the core focus of the Stillman Diet primarily revolves around macronutrient ratios, the importance of hydration cannot be overstated. Ensuring sufficient water intake is essential not only for supporting protein metabolism and overall health but also for addressing potential challenges arising from the dietary restrictions imposed by the Stillman Diet. Thus, prioritizing hydration emerges as a fundamental aspect of adherence to this or any other dietary plan, serving to optimize physiological functions and promote overall well-being.

The significance of water in the process of losing weight.

A comprehensive weight loss strategy recognizes the pivotal role of water as a fundamental component. Its significance transcends mere hydration, intricately weaving into a myriad of physiological processes that intricately influence metabolism, satiety, and overall well-being.

Primarily, optimal hydration is indispensable for maximizing metabolic efficiency. Adequate water intake facilitates the body's ability to convert stored carbohydrates and fats into energy, thereby enhancing metabolic function. Conversely, dehydration impedes metabolic processes, resulting in a sluggish metabolism that hampers calorie burning capacity.

Furthermore, water intake profoundly impacts appetite regulation and feelings of satiety. Pre-meal water consumption can promote a sense of fullness, potentially curbing calorie intake and aiding in weight management efforts. Moreover, proper hydration mitigates the risk of misinterpreting thirst cues as hunger, thereby averting unnecessary calorie consumption and impulsive snacking.

As a calorie-free beverage option, water serves as a strategic substitution for sugary and calorie-laden drinks, contributing to overall calorie reduction and creating a conducive environment for weight loss. Opting for water over calorific beverages not only slashes calorie intake but also supports the establishment of a calorie deficit, a cornerstone of successful weight loss endeavors.

Sustaining adequate hydration levels is equally paramount for optimizing physical performance during exercise, a crucial component of weight loss efforts. Dehydration can lead to fatigue and diminished exercise capacity, hindering the ability to engage in physical activity effectively and impeding calorie expenditure.

Moreover, water's involvement in thermogenesis underscores its role in calorie expenditure. Particularly when consumed cold, water prompts the body to expend additional energy to regulate its temperature, resulting in heightened calorie burning. This phenomenon accentuates water's multifaceted contribution to weight reduction efforts.

In essence, water emerges as a multifunctional ally in the pursuit of weight loss and overall health. Its role in regulating metabolism, promoting satiety, serving as a calorie-free beverage option, optimizing physical performance, and enhancing thermogenesis underscores its indispensability within a comprehensive weight loss regimen. Thus, prioritizing adequate hydration stands as a fundamental pillar of any effective weight management strategy, fostering optimal health outcomes and sustainable weight loss success.

Integrating Fluids into the Stillman Diet

Transitioning away from the Stillman Diet involves a multifaceted approach that encompasses not only adjustments in solid food intake but also careful consideration of fluid consumption. The Stillman Diet, renowned for its emphasis on carbohydrate restriction and ample protein intake, places a significant importance on maintaining hydration through adequate water and liquid intake. While much attention is often directed towards the solid components of meals, the role of liquids cannot be understated in ensuring the effectiveness and longevity of the diet plan.

Central to the principles of the Stillman Diet is the prioritization of water as the primary beverage choice. Sufficient hydration is vital for supporting various physiological processes, including digestion, nutrient absorption, and waste elimination. Given the diet's emphasis on heightened protein consumption, which can increase the body's water requirements, staying well-hydrated becomes particularly crucial to prevent dehydration and support optimal kidney function.

Moreover, maintaining adequate hydration levels plays a pivotal role in hunger management when adhering to a diet that restricts specific food categories. Consuming water before meals can promote a sense of fullness, potentially leading to reduced calorie intake overall—a strategy aligning with the Stillman Diet's objective of calorie control through protein-rich meals.

While water remains the cornerstone of hydration in the Stillman Diet, the plan does allow for the inclusion of additional low-calorie, carbohydrate-free beverages. Herbal teas, black coffee, and certain types of broth are among the permissible options, offering variety while adhering to the diet's carbohydrate limitations.

However, it is imperative to exercise caution with sugary and calorie-dense beverages, as these can undermine the metabolic state of ketosis—the primary goal of the Stillman Diet—by introducing excess calories and disrupting the body's fat-burning mechanisms.

In essence, liquids are an integral component of the Stillman Diet, serving not only to maintain hydration but also to support metabolism and appetite regulation. Choosing beverages that are low in calories and carbohydrates complements the foundational role of water in this dietary approach. Mindful selection of liquids aligns with the core tenets of the Stillman Diet and contributes to its sustained effectiveness. When incorporating liquids into the diet plan, individual preferences and tolerances should be taken into consideration, ensuring adherence and optimizing outcomes, as with any dietary regimen.

SECTION 5: LOW CARB RECIPES

STILLMAN DIET BREAKFAST RECIPES

Healthy pepper, tomato & ham omelette

Things Needed

2 whole eggs and 3 egg whites

1 tsp olive oil

1 red pepper, deseeded and finely chopped

2 spring onions, white and green parts kept separate, and finely chopped

few slices wafer-thin extra-lean ham, shredded

25g reduced-fat mature cheddar

wholemeal toast, to serve (optional)

1-2 chopped fresh tomatoes, to serve (optional)

Direction

STEP 1

Mix the eggs and egg whites with some seasoning and set aside. Heat the oil in a medium non-stick frying pan and cook the pepper for 3-4 mins. Throw in the white parts of the spring onions and cook for 1 min more. Pour in the eggs and cook over a medium heat until almost completely set.

STEP 2

Sprinkle on the ham and cheese, and continue cooking until just set in the centre, or flash it under a hot grill if you like it more well done. Serve straight from the pan with the green part of the spring onions sprinkled on top, the chopped tomato and some wholemeal toast, if you like.

Egg foo yung

Things Needed

2 tbsp groundnut oil

150g protein of choice, such as raw king prawns (de-shelled and de-veined) or cooked chicken, cooked char siu pork or pre-fried tofu, cut into bite-sized pieces

1 small white onion, cut into strips

40g sliced mushrooms

40g peas

¼ tsp white pepper

4 eggs, whisked

Direction

STEP 1

Heat a wok over a medium-high heat. Once hot, pour in the oil, then add your protein of choice and spread it out across the bottom of the wok. When it begins to brown, add the sliced onion and continue to cook for 1-2 mins, stirring regularly, to soften slightly. Tip in the mushrooms and stir.

STEP 2

When the mushrooms have started to soften, add the peas along with the white pepper and ½ tsp salt. Stir-fry for 1 min, then add the whisked eggs. Try not to stir the eggs – instead, pick up the wok and swirl the eggs around the rest of the Things Needed. Once they begin to set, slowly fold into the rest of the dish. Remove from the heat as soon as the eggs have nearly cooked all the way through.

Sweet poached egg

Things Needed

1 tbsp white wine vinegar

eggs, as many as you want to poach

Our Most Popular Alternative

Poached eggs with smashed avocado & tomatoes

Direction

STEP 1

Fill a large saucepan with water and add the vinegar. As soon as the water starts to boil, turn the heat down to a simmer.

STEP 2

Crack the egg into a small bowl. For a perfect egg with no wispy white bits, crack into a fine strainer and allow the runnier egg white to drain off.

STEP 3

Stir the water to create a gentle whirlpool which will help the egg white wrap around the yolk. Then carefully slide the egg into the water making sure the heat is low enough not to throw the egg around - there should only be small bubbles rising.

STEP 4

Cook for 3-4 mins, until the white is cooked through.

STEP 5

Remove gently using a slotted spoon and blot any water from the base on a tea towel or kitchen paper. You can add more than one egg to the pan but make sure each one has enough room.

Turkish one-pan eggs & peppers (Menemen)

Things Needed

2 tbsp olive oil

2 onions, sliced

1 red or green pepper, halved deseeded and sliced

1-2 red chillies, deseeded and sliced

400g can chopped tomatoes

1-2 tsp caster sugar

4 eggs

small bunch parsley, roughly chopped

6 tbsp thick, creamy yogurt

2 garlic cloves, crushed

Direction

STEP 1

Heat the oil in a heavy-based frying pan. Stir in the onions, pepper and chillies. Cook until they begin to soften. Add the tomatoes and sugar, mixing well. Cook until the liquid has reduced, season.

STEP 2

Using a wooden spoon, create 4 pockets in the tomato mixture and crack the eggs into them. Cover the pan and cook the eggs over a low heat until just set.

STEP 3

Beat the yogurt with the garlic and season. Sprinkle the menemen with parsley and serve from the frying pan with a dollop of the garlic-flavoured yogurt.

Courgette & ricotta fritters with poached eggs & harissa yogurt

Things Needed

2 courgettes, coarsely grated

50g ricotta

1⁄2 lemon, zested

2 eggs, lightly beaten

20g parmesan or vegetarian alternative, grated

50g self-raising flour

60g Greek yogurt

½ tbsp rose harissa

2 tbsp olive oil

6 thin slices of pancetta (optional)

splash of white wine vinegar

2 large eggs

dill and parsley, torn, to serve 8g

Direction

STEP 1

Line a bowl with a clean cloth and add the courgette with a pinch of salt. Set aside for 30 mins, then use the cloth to squeeze out the excess liquid. Tip the courgette into a bowl with the ricotta, lemon zest, eggs and parmesan, then stir to combine. Fold in the flour and some seasoning.

STEP 2

Stir the Greek yogurt and harissa together in a small bowl and season with a pinch of salt. Set aside.

STEP 3

Heat the oven to 180C/160C fan/gas 4. Heat the oil in a non-stick frying pan and spoon in six mounds of the courgette mixture. Cook over a medium heat for 3-4 mins each side until golden brown. Transfer to a baking sheet and bake for 10 mins.

STEP 4

Meanwhile, heat your grill to high, then cook the pancetta, if using, for 2-3 mins on each side until crisp.

STEP 5

Bring a pan of water to the boil. Drizzle a little of the vinegar into a ramekin and crack an egg into it. Swirl the water in the pan with a wooden spoon to create a whirlpool in the middle, then gently tip the egg into it and simmer for 3 mins. Repeat with the second egg. Serve three fritters stacked on each plate, topped with an egg and three slices of pancetta, alongside a dollop of the harissa yogurt, then scatter over the herbs.

Prawn tagliatelle with courgettes

Things Needed

2 tbsp olive oil

2 courgettes (about 500g), trimmed and coarsely grated

1 large garlic clove, finely grated

1 small red chilli, finely chopped

180g tagliatelle

150g raw king prawns, peeled and deveined

1 lemon, zested and juiced

½ small bunch of parsley, finely chopped

Direction

STEP 1

Heat the oil in a frying pan and fry the courgette for 4-5 mins, then stir through the garlic and chilli.

STEP 2

Cook the tagliatelle following pack instructions. Drain, reserving some of the cooking water.

STEP 3

Add the prawns to the courgette mixture, and cook for 2 mins until pink. Toss through the tagliatelle, the lemon zest and juice, parsley, some seasoning and a splash of the reserved cooking water. Divide between bowls and serve.

Chunky Bolognese soup with penne

Things Needed

2 tsp rapeseed oil

3 onions, finely chopped

3 large carrots, finely diced

2 celery sticks, finely diced

3 garlic cloves, finely chopped

250g pack 5% fat steak mince

500g carton passata

1 tbsp vegetable bouillon powder

1 tsp smoked paprika

4 sprigs fresh thyme

100g wholemeal penne

45g finely grated parmesan, plus extra to serve

Direction

STEP 1

Heat the oil in a large non-stick pan and fry the onions for a few mins. Add the carrots, celery and garlic, then fry for 5 mins, stirring until the vegetables start to soften.

STEP 2

Add the meat and stir well so it breaks down as it cooks. Once it's turned brown, add the passata and bouillon along with 1.3 litres of boiling water. Add the paprika, thyme and some black pepper. Cover the pan and simmer for 15 mins.

STEP 3

Tip in the penne and cook for 12-15 mins until tender. Stir through the cheese, then ladle into bowls. Sprinkle over extra cheese, if you like.

STEP 4

Cool the remaining soup, remove the thyme and chill. Will keep for up to seven days. Reheat in a pan, adding some water if it's thickened

Courgette & ricotta fritters with poached eggs & harissa yogurt

Things Needed

2 courgettes, coarsely grated

50g ricotta

1⁄2 lemon, zested

2 eggs, lightly beaten

20g parmesan or vegetarian alternative, grated

50g self-raising flour

60g Greek yogurt

1⁄2 tbsp rose harissa

2 tbsp olive oil

6 thin slices of pancetta (optional)

splash of white wine vinegar

2 large eggs

dill and parsley, torn, to serve 8g

Direction

STEP 1

Line a bowl with a clean cloth and add the courgette with a pinch of salt. Set aside for 30 mins, then use the cloth to squeeze out the excess liquid. Tip the courgette into a bowl with the ricotta, lemon zest, eggs and parmesan, then stir to combine. Fold in the flour and some seasoning.

STEP 2

Stir the Greek yogurt and harissa together in a small bowl and season with a pinch of salt. Set aside.

STEP 3

Heat the oven to 180C/160C fan/gas 4. Heat the oil in a non-stick frying pan and spoon in six mounds of the courgette mixture. Cook over a medium heat for 3-4 mins each side until golden brown. Transfer to a baking sheet and bake for 10 mins.

STEP 4

Meanwhile, heat your grill to high, then cook the pancetta, if using, for 2-3 mins on each side until crisp.

STEP 5

Bring a pan of water to the boil. Drizzle a little of the vinegar into a ramekin and crack an egg into it. Swirl the water in the pan with a wooden spoon to create a whirlpool in the middle, then gently tip the egg into it and simmer for 3 mins. Repeat with the second egg. Serve three fritters stacked on each plate, topped with an egg and three slices of pancetta, alongside a dollop of the harissa yogurt, then scatter over the herbs.

Breakfast pasta

Things Needed

For the pasta base

2 red onions, halved and thinly sliced

150g wholemeal penne

1 lemon, zested and juiced

1 tbsp rapeseed oil, plus a little extra for drizzling

2 large garlic cloves, finely grated

30g pack basil, chopped, stems and all

For the salmon pasta box

½ red pepper, sliced

1 salmon fillet

1 tsp capers

big handful rocket

For the chicken pasta box

1 large courgette, sliced

1 skinless chicken breast fillet, thickly sliced (150g)

2 tsp pesto

5 large cherry tomatoes, halved (80g)

For the aubergine pasta box

1 small aubergine, sliced then diced (about 275g)

5 large cherry tomatoes, quartered (80g)

5 kalamata olives, halved

Direction

STEP 1

Heat oven to 200C/180C fan/gas 6. Arrange the red onions, red pepper, courgette and aubergine in lines on a large baking sheet. Drizzle with a little oil and roast for 15 mins.

STEP 2

Cook the pasta for 10-12 mins until al dente. While the pasta is cooking, loosely wrap the

salmon fillet in foil and do the same with the
chicken and pesto in another foil parcel, then
put them on another baking tray.

STEP 3

When the veg have had their 15 mins, put the
salmon and chicken in the oven and cook for a
further 12 mins (or until the chicken is cooked
through). Drain the pasta, put in a bowl and
toss really well with the lemon zest and juice,
rapeseed oil, garlic and two-thirds of the basil.
When everything is cooked, add the red onions
to the pasta. Toss together and divide between
three lunch boxes.

STEP 4

Top the first box with the salmon fillet (remove
the skin first), then add the red pepper from the
tray. Scatter over the capers and add the rocket.

To the second box, add the chicken and pesto with any juices, the roasted courgette and the halved cherry tomatoes. In the third box, toss the aubergine into the pasta with the quartered cherry tomatoes, olives and the remaining basil. Seal up each container and chill. Eat within three days, preferably in the order of the salmon, then the chicken and then the aubergine.

STILLMAN DIET LUNCH RECIPES

Ratatouille

Things Needed

2 large aubergines

4 small courgettes

2 red or yellow peppers

4 large ripe tomatoes

5 tbsp olive oil

supermarket pack or small bunch basil

1 medium onion, peeled and thinly sliced

3 garlic cloves, peeled and crushed

1 tbsp red wine vinegar

1 tsp sugar (any kind)

Direction

STEP 1

Cut 2 large aubergines in half lengthways. Place them on the board, cut side down, slice in half lengthways again and then across into 1.5cm chunks. Cut the ends off 4 small courgettes, then across into 1.5cm slices.

STEP 2

Peel 2 red or yellow peppers from stalk to bottom. Hold upright, cut around the stalk, then cut into 3 pieces. Cut away any membrane, then chop into bite-size chunks.

STEP 3

Score a small cross on the base of each of 4 large ripe tomatoes, then put them into a heatproof bowl. Pour boiling water over, leave for 20 secs, then remove. Pour the water away, replace the tomatoes and cover with cold water. Leave to cool, then peel the skin away.

STEP 4

Quarter the tomatoes, scrape away the seeds with a spoon, then roughly chop the flesh.

STEP 5

Set a sauté pan over medium heat and when hot, pour in 2 tbsp olive oil. Brown the aubergines for 5 mins on each side until the pieces are soft. Set them aside.

STEP 6

Fry the courgettes in another tbsp oil for 5 mins, until golden on both sides. Repeat with the peppers. Don't overcook the vegetables at this stage.

STEP 7

Tear up the leaves from the bunch of basil and set aside. Cook 1 thinly sliced medium onion in the pan for 5 minutes. Add 3 crushed garlic cloves and fry for a further minute. Stir in 1 tbsp red wine vinegar and 1 tsp sugar, then tip in the tomatoes and half the basil.

STEP 8

Return the vegetables to the pan with some salt and pepper and cook for 5 mins. Serve with basil.

Chicken satay salad

Things Needed

1 tbsp tamari

1 tsp medium curry powder

¼ tsp ground cumin

1 garlic clove, finely grated

1 tsp clear honey

2 skinless chicken breast fillets (or use turkey breast)

1 tbsp crunchy peanut butter (choose a sugar-free version with no palm oil, if possible)

1 tbsp sweet chilli sauce

1 tbsp lime juice

sunflower oil, for wiping the pan

2 Little Gem lettuce hearts, cut into wedges

¼ cucumber, halved and sliced

1 banana shallot, halved and thinly sliced

coriander, chopped

seeds from ½ pomegranate

Direction

STEP 1

Pour the tamari into a large dish and stir in the curry powder, cumin, garlic and honey. Mix well. Slice the chicken breasts in half horizontally to make 4 fillets in total, then add to the marinade and mix well to coat. Set aside in the fridge for at least 1 hr, or overnight, to allow the flavours to penetrate the chicken.

STEP 2

Meanwhile, mix the peanut butter with the chilli sauce, lime juice, and 1 tbsp water to make a spoonable sauce. When ready to cook the chicken, wipe a large non-stick frying pan with a little oil. Add the chicken and cook, covered with a lid, for 5-6 mins on a medium heat, turning the fillets over for the last min, until cooked but still moist. Set aside, covered, to rest for a few mins.

STEP 3

While the chicken rests, toss the lettuce wedges with the cucumber, shallot, coriander and pomegranate, and pile onto plates. Spoon over a little sauce. Slice the chicken, pile on top of

the salad and spoon over the remaining sauce.
Eat while the chicken is still warm

Keralan chicken coconut ishtu

Things Needed

5 tbsp coconut oil or vegetable oil

5cm/2in cinnamon stick

6 green cardamom pods

4 cloves

10 black peppercorns, lightly crushed

1 star anise

15 curry leaves

1 medium onion, finely sliced

thumb-sized piece of ginger, peeled and finely chopped

6 garlic cloves, finely chopped

2-3 green chillies

2 tsp fennel seeds

½ tsp ground turmeric

1 tbsp ground coriander

600g chicken thighs, skinned

handful green beans, ends trimmed, halved if very long

400ml can coconut milk

2 tbsp coconut cream

1 tsp vinegar (or to taste)

large handful baby spinach, blanched and water squeezed out

small handful fresh coriander, to garnish

Direction

STEP 1

Heat the oil in a wide pan (a karahi or wok is ideal), then add the cinnamon stick, cardamom pods, cloves, peppercorns and star anise. Once the seeds have stopped popping, add the curry leaves and the onion and cook over a medium heat until translucent. Add the ginger, garlic and green chillies, and sauté gently for 1-2 mins or until the garlic is cooked.

STEP 2

Grind the fennel seeds to a fine powder in a spice grinder or with a pestle and mortar, then add to the pan with the turmeric, ground coriander and a pinch of salt. Add a splash of water and cook for 2 mins. Put the chicken in the pan and cook in the spice paste for 2 mins. Add water to come a third of the way up the chicken, bring to a boil, then reduce the heat and cook, covered, for 1 hr, stirring occasionally.

STEP 3

Once the liquid has reduced, add the green beans and coconut milk (including the thin milk that collects at the bottom of the can), cover and cook for another 10 mins. Uncover and cook off most of the excess liquid, stirring occasionally. Check the chicken is cooked all the way through. Stir in the coconut cream, vinegar and spinach, and bring to a simmer. Taste and adjust the seasoning, and serve topped with the coriande

Mediterranean turkey-stuffed peppers

Things Needed

2 red peppers (about 220g)

1 ½ tbsp olive oil, plus an extra drizzle

240g lean turkey breast mince (under 8% fat)

½ small onion, chopped

1 garlic clove, grated

1 tsp ground cumin

3-4 mushrooms, sliced

400g can chopped tomatoes

1 tbsp tomato purée

1 chicken stock cube

handful fresh oregano leaves

60g mozzarella, grated

150g green vegetables (spinach, kale, broccoli, mangetout or green beans), to serve

Direction

STEP 1

Heat oven to 190C/170C fan/gas 5. Halve the peppers lengthways, then remove the seeds and core but keep the stalks on. Rub the peppers with a drizzle of olive oil and season well. Put on a baking tray and roast for 15 mins.

STEP 2

Meanwhile, heat 1 tbsp olive oil in a large pan over a medium heat. Fry the mince for 2-3 mins, stirring to break up the chunks, then tip onto a plate.

STEP 3

Wipe out your pan, then heat the rest of the oil over a medium-high heat. Add the onion and garlic, stir-fry for 2-3 mins, then add the cumin and mushrooms and cook for 2-3 mins more.

STEP 4

Tip the mince back into the pan and add the chopped tomatoes and tomato purée. Crumble in the stock cube and cook for 3-4 mins, then add the oregano and season. Remove the peppers from the oven and fill them with as much of the mince as you can. (Don't worry if some spills out it – it will go satisfyingly crisp in the oven.) Top with the cheese and return to the oven for 10-15 mins until the cheese starts to turn golden.

STEP 5

Carefully slide the peppers onto a plate and serve alongside a pile of your favourite greens blanched, boiled or steamed.

Epic summer salad

Things Needed

400g black beans, drained

2 large handfuls baby spinach leaves, roughly chopped

500g heritage tomatoes, chopped into large chunks

½ cucumber, halved lengthways, seeds scooped out and sliced on an angle

1 mango, peeled and chopped into chunks

1 large red onion, halved and finely sliced

6-8 radishes, sliced

2 avocados, peeled and sliced

100g feta, crumbled

handful of herbs (reserved from the dressing)

For the dressing

large bunch mint

small bunch coriander

small bunch basil

1 fat green chilli, deseeded and chopped

1 small garlic clove

100ml extra virgin olive oil or rapeseed oil

2 limes, zested and juiced

2 tbsp white wine vinegar

2 tsp honey

Direction

STEP 1

Make the dressing by blending all of the Things Needed in a food processor (or very finely chop them), saving a few herb leaves for the salad. You can make the dressing up to 24 hrs before serving.

STEP 2

Scatter the beans and spinach over a large platter. Arrange the tomatoes, cucumber, mango, onion and radishes on top and gently toss together with your hands. Top the salad with the avocados, feta and herbs, and serve the dressing on the side

One-pot coconut fish curry

Things Needed

1 tbsp oil

1 onion, chopped

1 large garlic clove, crushed

1 tsp turmeric

1 tsp garam masala

1 tsp chilli flakes

400ml can coconut milk

390g pack fish pie mix

200g frozen peas

1 lime, cut into wedges

yogurt and rice (or cauliflower rice), to serve

Direction

STEP 1

Heat the oil in a large saucepan over a medium heat, add the onion and a big pinch of salt. Gently fry until the onion is translucent, so around 10 mins, then add the garlic and spices. Stir and cook for another minute, adding a splash of water to prevent them sticking. Tip in the coconut milk and stir well, then simmer for 10 mins.

STEP 2

Tip the fish pie mix and the frozen peas into the pan and cook until the peas are bright green and the fish is starting the flake, so around 3 mins. Season and add lime juice to taste. Ladle into bowls and serve with yogurt and rice.

Old Delhi-style butter chicken

Things Needed

800g boneless and skinless chicken thighs, cut into bite-sized pieces

coriander leaves, finely sliced red onion, sliced green or red chilli, naan bread or basmati rice, and chutney, to serve

For the marinade

120g Greek yogurt

thumb-sized piece ginger, grated

4-5 garlic cloves, crushed

1 tbsp vegetable or coconut oil

1 lemon, juiced

3 tsp mild chilli powder

1 tsp ground cumin

½ tsp garam masala

½ tsp turmeric

For the sauce

1kg ripe vine or plum tomatoes

thumb-sized piece ginger, peeled, half grated and half finely chopped

4 garlic cloves, crushed

4 green cardamom pods

2 cloves

1 bay leaf

1-2 tsp chilli powder

80g butter, diced

2 green chillies, cut lengthways

75ml single cream, plus a drizzle to serve

5-6 dried fenugreek leaves, crushed between your fingers (optional)

1 tsp garam masala

1 tbsp sugar or xylitol

For the spiced butter (optional)

3 tbsp ghee (see below) or butter

2 tsp black mustard seeds

1 dried whole Kashmiri chilli

6-8 dried curry leaves

Direction

STEP 1

Mix all of the marinade Things Needed together in a large mixing bowl with 1½ tsp salt. Add the chicken pieces and mix together until well-coated, then cover the bowl and chill for 1 hr or overnight in the fridge.

STEP 2

Heat the oven to 240C/220C fan/gas 9. Transfer the chicken pieces to a large baking tray (discard any remaining marinade), and cook for 10-15 mins. Turn the pieces after 10 mins so they colour evenly on both sides. The chicken doesn't need to be completely cooked through at this point as it will cook for a few more mins in the sauce.

STEP 3

Meanwhile, for the sauce, slice the tomatoes in half and put in a large pan in a single layer with 125ml water, the grated ginger, garlic, cardamom, cloves and bay leaf. Simmer, covered, until the tomatoes have completely disintegrated, about 20-25 mins. Remove the whole spices and blend the tomato mixture with a stick blender, then pass it through a sieve to make a smooth purée. Return to a clean pan, add the chilli powder and simmer for 12-15 mins. It should slowly begin to thicken. When the sauce turns glossy, add the chicken pieces and any of the reserved roasting juices from the tray.

STEP 4

Slowly stir in the butter, a couple of pieces at a time, and simmer for 6-8 mins until the chicken is cooked through. Add the chopped ginger, green chillies and cream, then simmer for a min or two longer, taking care that the sauce doesn't split. Stir in 1 tsp salt, fenugreek leaves, if using, and the garam masala, then check the seasoning, adjust if necessary, then add the sugar. In a separate pan, warm all the Things Needed for the spiced butter, if using, until the seeds start to pop (see below). Spoon over the curry, scatter with the coriander, onion, chilli, and a drizzle more cream, if using. Serve with naan, pilau rice and chutney or keto bread for a keto-friendly version.

Baked Salmon & Leek parcel

Things Needed

250g leek (about 3 small ones), thinly sliced

85g mascarpone

1 tbsp chopped dill, plus 1 tsp

2 skinless salmon fillets

½ lemon, grated zest of 1/4, plus a good squeeze of juice

2-3 tsp capers

spinach wilted, to serve (optional)

Direction

STEP 1

Heat oven to 200C/180C fan/gas 6. Place two sheets of baking parchment (large enough to wrap up each salmon fillet) on your work surface.

STEP 2

Put the leeks in a pan with 6 tbsp water, cover and bring to the boil. Cook for 5 mins until the water has been absorbed and the leeks are almost tender. Stir in the mascarpone, 1 tbsp dill and some seasoning.

STEP 3

Spoon half the creamy leeks into the middle of one sheet of parchment and place a salmon fillet on top, then repeat to make a second parcel. Sprinkle over the lemon zest with a squeeze of juice, then scatter over the capers and the remaining 1 tsp dill.

STEP 4

Bring the parchment up over the fish and join the two edges together by folding them over several times down the middle. Do the same with the ends and place the parcels, spaced apart, on a baking sheet.

STEP 5

Bake for 12-15 mins, depending on how well done you like your fish, then carefully tear open the parcel. Serve with lemon wedges for squeezing over and wilted spinach, if you like.

Sea bass with braised courgettes

Things Needed

2 tbsp extra virgin olive oil

1 thyme sprig

2 sea bass fillets

½ lemon, juiced

For the braised courgettes

4 tbsp extra virgin olive oil

pinch of fennel seeds

1 red onion, finely sliced

pinch of dried red chilli

handful of cherry tomatoes, cut in half

1 garlic clove, peeled and finely chopped

2 medium or 1 large courgette (about 200g), sliced 0.5cm thick

100ml white wine or sherry

1 lemon, juiced, plus extra wedges to serve

handful of dill, chopped

For the harissa mayo

4 tbsp good-quality, shop-bought mayonnaise

1 tbsp harissa, or more, to taste

Direction

STEP 1

Stir the mayonnaise and harissa together and refrigerate until ready to use.

STEP 2

For the courgettes, heat the olive oil in a high-sided, non-stick frying pan over a medium-high heat. Cook the fennel seeds, red onion and chilli with a pinch of salt for 5 mins until softened and fragrant. Add the cherry tomatoes, garlic and courgette, then season and cook down for a few mins. Pour in the wine, lemon juice and about 200ml water and simmer for 15-20 mins until the tomatoes and courgettes are collapsing. Bubble off any excess water. Stir through the dill and keep warm while you cook the sea bass. (Take your fish out of the fridge 20 mins before you cook it to bring it up to room temperature.)

STEP 3

Heat the olive oil with the thyme in a non-stick frying pan over a low-to-medium heat. Place the sea bass fillets skin-side down in the pan.

Season the flesh-side of the fillets with salt and pepper. Cook gently for about 8 mins until the skin is crisp (it might spit during this time, so best to wear an apron), then add a small amount of lemon juice and baste the flesh of the fish in the warm oil and lemon for about 4 mins, or until opaque and cooked through.

STEP 4

Divide the vegetables between plates and top with the bass. Serve with the harissa mayo and lemon wedges

Ginger & soy salmon en papillote

Things Needed

2 tbsp light soy sauce

1 tbsp rice wine vinegar

thumb-sized piece of ginger, finely grated

1 garlic clove, finely grated

2 skinless salmon fillets (about 140g each)

1 courgette, ends trimmed and spiralized into thin noodles

1 carrot, peeled, ends trimmed and spiralized into thin noodles

2 bulbs of pak choi (about 200g), leaves separated

1 red chilli, thinly sliced, deseeded if you like

Thai cauliflower rice, to serve (optional)

Direction

STEP 1

Heat oven to 180C/160C fan/gas 4. Before you prep the veg mix together the soy, vinegar, ginger, garlic and some black pepper in a bowl. Add the salmon fillets, cover and leave to marinate for 10 mins at room temperature or up to 2 hrs in the fridge.

STEP 2

Tear two large sheets of baking parchment, big enough to encase the fish and vegetables in and put onto a baking tray.

STEP 3

Divide the vegetables between the centre of the paper and top each with a marinated salmon fillet and the sliced chilli. Bring the sides of the parchment up over the salmon and pour half of the remaining marinade over each fillet then scrunch the paper tightly together to seal the fish in a parcel.

STEP 4

Roast for 20–25 mins, until the salmon is just cooked through and flakes into large pieces. Serve the fish in the parcel with some cauliflower or regular rice, if you like.

Superhealthy salmon burgers

Things Needed

4 boneless, skinless salmon fillets, about 550g/1lb 4oz in total, cut into chunks

2 tbsp Thai red curry paste

thumb-size piece fresh root ginger, grated

1 tsp soy sauce

1 bunch coriander, half chopped, half leaves picked

1 tsp vegetable oil

lemon wedges, to serve

For the salad

2 carrots

half large or 1 small cucumber

2 tbsp white wine vinegar

1 tsp golden caster sugar

Direction

STEP 1

Tip the salmon into a food processor with the paste, ginger, soy and chopped coriander. Pulse until roughly minced. Tip out the mix and shape into 4 burgers. Heat the oil in a non-stick frying pan, then fry the burgers for 4-5 mins on each side, turning until crisp and cooked through.

STEP 2

Meanwhile, use a swivel peeler to peel strips of carrot and cucumber into a bowl. Toss with the vinegar and sugar until the sugar has dissolved, then toss through the coriander leaves. Divide the salad between 4 plates. Serve with the burgers and rice.

Spicy meatballs with chilli black beans

Things Needed

1 red onion, halved and sliced

2 garlic cloves, sliced

1 large yellow pepper, quartered, deseeded and diced

1 tsp ground cumin

2-3 tsp chipotle chilli paste

300ml reduced-salt chicken stock

400g can cherry tomatoes

400g can black beans or red kidney beans, drained

1 avocado, stoned, peeled and chopped

juice ½ lime

For the meatballs

500g pack turkey breast mince

50g porridge oats

2 spring onions, finely chopped

1 tsp ground cumin

1 tsp coriander

small bunch coriander, chopped, stalks and leaves kept separate

1 tsp rapeseed oil

Direction

STEP 1

First make the meatballs. Tip the mince into a bowl, add the oats, spring onions, spices and the coriander stalks, then lightly knead the Things Needed together until well mixed. Shape into 12 ping-pong- sized balls. Heat the oil in a non-stick frying pan, add the meatballs and cook, turning them frequently, until golden. Remove from the pan.

STEP 2

Tip the onion and garlic into the pan with the pepper and stir-fry until softened. Stir in the cumin and chilli paste, then pour in the stock. Return the meatballs to the pan and cook, covered, over a low heat for 10 mins. Stir in the tomatoes and beans, and cook, uncovered, for a few mins more. Toss the avocado chunks in the lime juice and serve the meatballs topped with the avocado and coriander leaves.

Lentil bolognese

Things Needed

3 tbsp olive oil

2 onions, finely chopped

3 carrots, finely chopped

3 celery sticks, finely chopped

3 garlic cloves, crushed

500g bag dried red lentils

2 x 400g cans chopped tomatoes

2 tbsp tomato purée

2 tsp each dried oregano and thyme

3 bay leaves

1l vegetable stock

500g spaghetti

parmesan or vegetarian cheese, grated, to serve

Direction

STEP 1

Heat the oil in a large saucepan and add the onions, carrots, celery and garlic. Cook gently for 15-20 mins until everything is softened. Stir in the lentils, chopped tomatoes, tomato purée, herbs and stock. Bring to a simmer, then cook for 40-50 mins until the lentils are tender and saucy – splash in water if you need. Season.

STEP 2

If eating straight away, keep on a low heat while you cook the spaghetti, following pack instructions. Drain well, divide between pasta bowls or plates, spoon sauce over the top and grate over some cheese. Alternatively, cool the sauce and chill for up to 3 days. Or freeze for up to 3 months. Simply defrost portions overnight at room temperature, then reheat gently to serve.

Seafood rice

Things Needed

1 tbsp olive oil

1 leek or onion, sliced

110g pack chorizo sausage, chopped

1 tsp turmeric

300g long grain rice

1l hot fish or chicken stock

200g frozen peas

400g frozen seafood mix, defrosted

Direction

STEP 1

Heat the oil in a deep frying pan, then soften the leek for 5 mins without browning. Add the chorizo and fry until it releases its oils. Stir in the turmeric and rice until coated by the oils, then pour in the stock. Bring to the boil, then simmer for 15 mins, stirring occasionally.

STEP 2

Tip in the peas and cook for 5 mins, then stir in the seafood to heat through for a final 1-2 mins cooking or until rice is cooked. Check for seasoning and serve immediately with lemon wedges

Sesame salmon, purple sprouting broccoli & sweet potato mash

Things Needed

1 ½ tbsp sesame oil

1 tbsp low-salt soy sauce

thumb-sized piece ginger, grated

1 garlic clove, crushed

1 tsp honey

2 sweet potatoes, scrubbed and cut into wedges

1 lime, cut into wedges

2 boneless skinless salmon fillets

250g purple sprouting broccoli

1 tbsp sesame seeds

1 red chilli, thinly sliced (deseeded if you don't like it too hot)

Direction

STEP 1

Heat oven to 200C/180 fan/ gas 6 and line a baking tray with parchment. Mix together 1/2 tbsp sesame oil, the soy, ginger, garlic and honey. Put the sweet potato wedges, skin and all, into a glass bowl with the lime wedges. Cover with cling film and microwave on high for 12-14 mins until completely soft.

STEP 2

Meanwhile, spread the broccoli and salmon out on the baking tray. Spoon over the marinade and season. Roast in the oven for 10-12 mins, then sprinkle over the sesame seeds.

STEP 3

Remove the lime wedges and roughly mash the sweet potato using a fork. Mix in the remaining sesame oil, the chilli and some seasoning. Divide between plates, along with the salmon and broccoli.

Prawn tagliatelle with courgettes

Things Needed

2 tbsp olive oil

2 courgettes (about 500g), trimmed and coarsely grated

1 large garlic clove, finely grated

1 small red chilli, finely chopped

180g tagliatelle

150g raw king prawns, peeled and deveined

1 lemon, zested and juiced

½ small bunch of parsley, finely chopped

Direction

STEP 1

Heat the oil in a frying pan and fry the courgette for 4-5 mins, then stir through the garlic and chilli.

STEP 2

Cook the tagliatelle following pack instructions. Drain, reserving some of the cooking water.

STEP 3

Add the prawns to the courgette mixture, and cook for 2 mins until pink. Toss through the tagliatelle, the lemon zest and juice, parsley, some seasoning and a splash of the reserved cooking water. Divide between bowls and serve.

Chicken & lemon skewers

Things Needed

1 small pack mint, leaves picked

150g natural yogurt, plus extra to serve (optional)

1 lemon, zested and juiced

½ tsp ground cumin

½ tsp ground coriander

2cm piece ginger, grated

4 skinless chicken breasts, each cut into 6 pieces

4 wholemeal flatbreads or pittas

2 Little Gem lettuces, sliced

1 small red onion, sliced, to serve

pickled red cabbage, chilli sauce and hummus, to serve (all optional)

You will need

4 metal or wooden skewers

Direction

STEP 1

Chop half the mint and put in a bowl with the yogurt, half the lemon juice, all the lemon zest, spices and ginger. Mix well and season with lots of black pepper and a pinch of salt. Add the chicken pieces, mix well and put in the fridge for 20-30 mins. Meanwhile, soak 4 large wooden skewers in water for at least 20 mins (or use metal ones).

STEP 2

When you're ready to cook the chicken, heat your grill to a medium heat and line the grill tray with foil. Thread the chicken onto the soaked wooden or metal skewers and grill for 15-20 mins, turning halfway through, until browned and cooked through.

STEP 3

Warm the flatbreads under the grill for a couple of seconds, then serve them topped with the lettuce, chicken, red onion, remaining lemon juice and mint, and any optional extras such as extra yogurt or pickled cabbage, chilli sauce and hummus.

Slow cooker lamb curry

Things Needed

1 large onion, halved and sliced

3 tbsp Madras curry paste

400g can chopped tomatoes

2 tsp vegetable bouillon powder

25g red lentils

210g can chickpeas (don't drain)

1 tbsp grated ginger

1 tsp cumin seeds

1 cinnamon stick

75g curly kale

2 lean lamb steaks, fat removed, diced (about 240g)

cooked brown rice, to serve

Direction

STEP 1

Put all of the Things Needed into the slow cooker pot with a third of a can of water and stir well. Cover with the lid and chill in the fridge overnight.

STEP 2

The next day, stir again, then cook on Low for 6 hrs until the lamb and vegetables are tender. Serve with brown rice.

Spicy chicken & avocado wraps

Things Needed

1 chicken breast (approx 180g), thinly sliced at an angle

generous squeeze juice 0.5 lime

½ tsp mild chilli powder

1 garlic clove, chopped

1 tsp olive oil

2 seeded wraps

1 avocado, halved and stoned

1 roasted red pepper from a jar, sliced

a few sprigs coriander, chopped

Direction

STEP 1

Mix the chicken with the lime juice, chilli powder and garlic.

STEP 2

Heat the oil in a non-stick frying pan then fry the chicken for a couple of mins – it will cook very quickly so keep an eye on it. Meanwhile, warm the wraps following the pack instructions or, if you have a gas hob, heat them over the flame to slightly char them. Do not let them dry out or they are difficult to roll.

STEP 3

Squash half an avocado onto each wrap, add the peppers to the pan to warm them through then pile onto the wraps with the chicken, and sprinkle over the coriander. Roll up, cut in half and eat with your fingers.

STILLMAN DIET DINNER RECIPES

Sesame salmon, purple sprouting broccoli & sweet potato mash

Things Needed

1 ½ tbsp sesame oil

1 tbsp low-salt soy sauce

thumb-sized piece ginger, grated

1 garlic clove, crushed

1 tsp honey

2 sweet potatoes, scrubbed and cut into wedges

1 lime, cut into wedges

2 boneless skinless salmon fillets

250g purple sprouting broccoli

1 tbsp sesame seeds

1 red chilli, thinly sliced (deseeded if you don't like it too hot)

Direction

STEP 1

Heat oven to 200C/180 fan/ gas 6 and line a baking tray with parchment. Mix together 1/2 tbsp sesame oil, the soy, ginger, garlic and honey. Put the sweet potato wedges, skin and all, into a glass bowl with the lime wedges. Cover with cling film and microwave on high for 12-14 mins until completely soft.

STEP 2

Meanwhile, spread the broccoli and salmon out on the baking tray. Spoon over the marinade and season. Roast in the oven for 10-12 mins, then sprinkle over the sesame seeds.

STEP 3

Remove the lime wedges and roughly mash the sweet potato using a fork. Mix in the remaining sesame oil, the chilli and some seasoning. Divide between plates, along with the salmon and broccoli.

Chicken stroganoff

Things Needed

2 tbsp olive oil

4 skinless chicken breasts, cut into chunks

2 onions, finely chopped

4 garlic cloves, crushed

1 tbsp sweet paprika

400ml chicken stock

4 tsp Dijon mustard

2 tbsp Worcestershire sauce

200g soured cream or crème fraiche

a large handful of parsley, chopped

rice mash or pasta, to serve

Direction

STEP 1

Heat half the oil in a frying pan and fry the chicken pieces over a medium high heat, stirring frequently. until golden brown. Season and transfer to a plate.

STEP 2

Heat the remaining oil and lower the heat to medium. Fry the onion for 6-8 mins until softened but not golden, then stir in the garlic and paprika. Fry for a minute until fragrant, then pour in the stock, and add the Dijon and Worcestershire sauce. Tip in the seared chicken with any resting juices, and simmer for 5-6 mins until reduced slightly and the chicken is cooked through.

STEP 3

Over a low heat, stir in the soured cream until just combined to create a creamy sauce, and it's just started to simmer. Scatter over the parsley and serve with rice, mash or pasta, if you like.

Vegetarian ramen

Things Needed

80g pack instant noodles (look for an Asian brand with a flavour like sesame)

2 spring onions, finely chopped

½ head pak choi

1 egg

1 tsp sesame seeds

chilli sauce, to serve

Direction

STEP 1

Cook the noodles with the sachet of flavouring provided (or use stock instead of the sachet, if you have it). Add the spring onions and pak choi for the final min.

STEP 2

Meanwhile, simmer the egg for 6 mins from boiling, run it under cold water to stop it cooking, then peel it. Toast the sesame seeds in a frying pan.

STEP 3

Tip the noodles and greens into a deep bowl, halve the boiled egg and place on top. Sprinkle with sesame seeds, then drizzle with the sauce or sesame oil provided with the noodles, and chilli sauce, if using.

Easy butter chicken

Things Needed

500g skinless boneless chicken thighs

For the marinade

1/2-1 lemon, (to taste) juiced

2 tsp ground cumin

2 tsp paprika

1-2 tsp hot chilli powder

200g natural yogurt

For the curry

2 tbsp vegetable oil

1 large onion, chopped

3 garlic cloves, crushed

1 green chilli, deseeded and finely chopped (optional)

thumb-sized piece ginger, grated

1 tsp garam masala

2 tsp ground fenugreek

3 tbsp tomato purée

300ml chicken stock

50g flaked almonds, toasted

To serve (optional)

cooked basmati rice

naan bread

mango chutney or lime pickle

fresh coriander

lime wedges

Direction

STEP 1

In a medium bowl, mix all the marinade Things Needed with some seasoning. Chop the chicken into bite-sized pieces and toss with the marinade. Cover and chill in the fridge for 1 hr or overnight.

STEP 2

In a large, heavy saucepan, heat the oil. Add the onion, garlic, green chilli, ginger and some seasoning. Fry on a medium heat for 10 mins or until soft.

STEP 3

Add the spices with the tomato purée, cook for a further 2 mins until fragrant, then add the stock and marinated chicken. Cook for 15 mins, then add any remaining marinade left in the bowl. Simmer for 5 mins, then sprinkle with the toasted almonds. Serve with rice, naan bread, chutney, coriander and lime wedges, if you like.

Prawn jambalaya

Things Needed

1 tbsp rapeseed oil

1 onion, chopped

3 celery sticks, sliced

100g wholegrain basmati rice

1 tsp mild chilli powder

1 tbsp ground coriander

½ tsp fennel seeds

400g can chopped tomatoes

1 tsp vegetable bouillon powder

1 yellow pepper, roughly chopped

2 garlic cloves, chopped

1 tbsp fresh thyme leaves

150g pack small prawns, thawed if frozen

3 tbsp chopped parsley

Direction

STEP 1

Heat the oil in a large, deep frying pan. Add the onion and celery, and fry for 5 mins to soften. Add the rice and spices, and pour in the tomatoes with just under 1 can of water. Stir in the bouillon powder, pepper, garlic and thyme.

STEP 2

Cover the pan with a lid and simmer for 30 mins until the rice is tender and almost all the liquid has been absorbed. Stir in the prawns and parsley, cook briefly to heat through, then serve.

Slow cooker bolognese

Things Needed

4 tbsp olive oil

6 smoked bacon rashers, chopped

1½kg lean minced beef (or use half beef, half pork mince)

4 onions, finely chopped

3 carrots, finely chopped

4 celery sticks, finely chopped

8 garlic cloves, crushed

500g mushrooms, sliced

4 x 400g cans chopped tomatoes

6 tbsp tomato purée

2 tbsp dried mixed herbs

2 bay leaves

large glass red wine (optional)

4 tbsp red wine vinegar

1 tbsp sugar

cooked spaghetti, to serve

parmesan, to serve

Direction

STEP 1

Heat the oil in a large pan and fry the bacon and mince in batches until browned. Add to the slow cooker.

STEP 2

Add the onions, carrots, celery, garlic, mushrooms, tomatoes, tomato purée, herbs, wine (if using), vinegar, sugar and seasoning to the slow cooker. Cover and cook on Low for 6-8 hours, then uncover, turn to High and cook for another hour until thick and saucy.

STEP 3

Serve with cooked spaghetti and grated or shaved parmesan

Sweet Chicken 65

Things Needed

1½ tsp cumin seeds

750g skinless and boneless chicken thighs

120g Greek-style yogurt

2 tbsp lime juice

2 tbsp grated ginger

5 large garlic cloves, finely grated

1 tbsp finely chopped curry leaves

1 tbsp finely chopped coriander leaves

1½ tbsp deggi mirch spice blend

1 tsp amchoor powder (dried green mango powder, optional)

½ tsp sugar

3 tbsp rapeseed oil

1 tbsp tomato ketchup

3 tbsp rice flour

vegetable oil, for deep-frying

3 green chillies, slit lengthwise

1 tbsp finely chopped garlic

generous handful of whole curry leaves

lime wedges, to serve

Direction

STEP 1

Dry-toast the cumin seeds in a small frying pan over a medium heat. Cool then put in a coffee or spice grinder and grind into a fine powder. Set aside. Cut the chicken thighs into quarters and combine in a mixing bowl with the yogurt, lime juice and 1½ tsp salt. Mix well. Mix in the grated ginger, garlic, 1 tsp ground black pepper, chopped curry leaves, chopped coriander, deggi mirch, amchoor powder (if using), sugar, 1 tbsp of the rapeseed oil and tomato ketchup. Mix well to ensure all the chicken pieces are thoroughly coated. Cover the bowl with and keep chilled for 3 hrs.

STEP 2

Remove the chicken from the fridge and leave for 30 mins. Stir in the rice flour and the roasted cumin powder mixture from step 1, and stir well.

STEP 3

Fill a large pan three-quarters full with oil and heat to 180C or until the batter sizzles when a little is dropped in. Take each piece of chicken individually and gently slide into the pan. Take care not to cook too many pieces in one go. The pieces should be bubbling when in the oil. Allow to cook for 3-4 mins, then carefully remove with a slotted spoon and drain on a plate lined with kitchen paper. Repeat for all the chicken pieces and set aside.

STEP 4

Put the remaining 2 tbsp rapeseed oil in a wok or karai and heat over a medium-high heat. Add the slit chillies, chopped garlic and curry leaves. Take care as the Things Needed may pop. Cook for 1 min, then add the fried chicken and gently toss. Stir well for another minute to coat the chicken. Remove from the heat and serve with lime wedges on the side.

Moroccan chicken stew

Things Needed

large handful flaked almonds

1 tbsp ghee

2 red onions, finely sliced

4 garlic cloves, finely chopped

thumb-sized piece ginger (about 40g), unpeeled if organic, finely grated

1 tsp ground cumin

1 tsp ground cinnamon

½ smoked sweet paprika

4 chicken thighs, skin on

2 red peppers, sliced into thin strips

1 large lemon, cut into 6 thick slices

handful green olives, stoned

250ml gluten-free chicken stock or bone broth

4 pitted dates or dried apricots, chopped

a small pinch of chilli powder or 1 fresh, red chilli, chopped (optional)

150g green beans, halved

handful fresh coriander, chopped

handful fresh parsley, chopped

Direction

STEP 1

In a large, dry pan, gently toast the almonds for 2 mins until golden – don't take your eyes off them, as they burn easily – then set aside.

STEP 2

In the same pan, heat the ghee and gently cook the onions for 8 mins until softened. Add the garlic, ginger and spices, and fry for 1 min more.

STEP 3

Add the chicken thighs, skin-side down, and cook until the skin is golden and crisp, then turn and cook to lightly golden on the flesh side.

STEP 4

Add the red peppers, lemon slices, olives, stock or bone broth and dates or apricots (and chilli, if using). Simmer with the lid on for about 40 mins until the chicken is cooked through.

STEP 5

If you find the sauce is too watery, take off the lid and leave it to reduce a little. If the sauce is too thick, add a few more tbsps of water.

STEP 6

Add the green beans for the final 4 mins of cooking time. Season to taste and top with the coriander, parsley and the toasted almonds to serve.

Vegan chickpea curry jacket potatoes

Things Needed

4 sweet potatoes

1 tbsp coconut oil

1 ½ tsp cumin seeds

1 large onion, diced

2 garlic cloves, crushed

thumb-sized piece ginger, finely grated

1 green chilli, finely chopped

1 tsp garam masala

1 tsp ground coriander

½ tsp turmeric

2 tbsp tikka masala paste

2 x 400g can chopped tomatoes

2 x 400g can chickpeas, drained

lemon wedges and coriander leaves, to serve

Direction

STEP 1

Heat oven to 200C/180C fan/gas 6. Prick the sweet potatoes all over with a fork, then put on a baking tray and roast in the oven for 45 mins or until tender when pierced with a knife.

STEP 2

Meanwhile, melt the coconut oil in a large saucepan over medium heat. Add the cumin seeds and fry for 1 min until fragrant, then add the onion and fry for 7-10 mins until softened.

STEP 3

Put the garlic, ginger and green chilli into the pan, and cook for 2-3 mins. Add the spices and tikka masala paste and cook for a further 2 mins until fragrant, then tip in the tomatoes. Bring to a simmer, then tip in the chickpeas and cook for a further 20 mins until thickened. Season.

STEP 4

Put the roasted sweet potatoes on four plates and cut open lengthways. Spoon over the chickpea curry and squeeze over the lemon wedges. Season, then scatter with coriander before serving

Curried spinach, eggs & chickpeas

Things Needed

1 tbsp rapeseed oil

1 onion, thinly sliced

1 garlic clove, crushed

3cm piece ginger, peeled and grated

1 tsp ground turmeric

1 tsp ground coriander

1 tsp garam masala

1 tbsp ground cumin

450g tomatoes, chopped

400g can chickpeas, drained

1 tsp sugar

200g spinach

2 large eggs

3 tbsp natural yogurt

1 red chilli, finely sliced

½ small bunch of coriander, torn

Direction

STEP 1

Heat the oil in a large frying pan or flameproof casserole pot over a medium heat, and fry the onion for 10 mins until golden and sticky. Add the garlic, ginger, turmeric, ground coriander, garam masala, cumin and tomatoes, and fry for 2 mins more. Add the chickpeas, 100ml water and the sugar and bring to a simmer. Stir in the spinach, then cover and cook for 20-25 mins. Season to taste.

STEP 2

Cook the eggs in a pan of boiling water for 7 mins, then rinse under cold running water to cool. Drain, peel and halve. Swirl the yogurt into the curry, then top with the eggs, chilli and coriander. Season.

Delicious Khatti dhal

Things Needed

For the dhal

430g toor dhal or red split lentils

½ tsp turmeric

2 large tomatoes, chopped (better if you remove the skin but not essential)

5cm piece ginger, peeled and grated

2 garlic cloves, crushed or grated

2 green chillies, chopped (deseeded if you don't like it very hot)

2 tbsp tamarind paste

1 tsp hot chilli powder

2 tsp ground coriander

For the tempering

2 tbsp oil or ghee (or a mixture of oil and unsalted butter)

½ tsp cumin seeds

8 garlic cloves, sliced

3 dried chillies (I use Kashmiri), roughly broken

12 curry leaves, fresh or frozen (optional)

Direction

STEP 1

Soak the toor dhal for about 40 mins, then rinse well. Put it in a large heavy-bottomed saucepan with the turmeric, tomatoes, ginger, garlic and chillies. Add 1.7 litres of water and bring to the boil. Turn the heat down low and cook until you have a thick purée, adding water if it gets too dry. Dhal can be quite soupy or quite thick, depending on how you like it. Simply reduce it to thicken it, or add water to thin it. Season to taste.

STEP 2

When the dhal is at a thickness you like, add the tamarind, chilli powder (unless it's already hot enough), and the ground coriander and check the seasoning.

STEP 3

Tempering is the last phase for a dhal. Heat the oil or ghee in a frying pan and add the cumin seeds. Cook over a medium heat for about 30 secs, then add the garlic and cook for about 10 secs (the garlic should eventually become golden but not brown so don't overdo it at this point), then add the dried chillies and the curry leaves, if using. Fry until the dried chillies have changed colour slightly and the curry leaves are crisp. Pour this over the dhal and stir. Cover and leave to sit for a few mins before serving.

Big-batch bolognese

Things Needed

4 tbsp olive oil

6 smoked bacon rashers, chopped

4 onions, finely chopped

3 carrots, finely chopped

4 celery sticks, finely chopped

8 garlic cloves, crushed

2 tbsp dried mixed herbs

2 bay leaves

500g mushrooms, sliced

1½ kg lean minced beef (or use half beef, half pork mince)

6 x 400g cans chopped tomatoes

6 tbsp tomato purée

large glass red wine (optional)

4 tbsp red wine vinegar

1 tbsp sugar

parmesan, to serve

Direction

STEP 1

Heat the oil in a very large saucepan. Gently cook the bacon, onions, carrots and celery for 20 mins until golden. Add the garlic, herbs, bay and mushrooms, then cook for 2 mins more.

STEP 2

Heat a large frying pan until really hot. Crumble in just enough mince to cover the pan, cook until brown, then tip in with the veg. Continue to fry the mince in batches until used up. Tip the tomatoes and purée in with the mince and veg. Rinse the cans out with the red wine, if you have some, or with a little water, then add to the pan with the vinegar and sugar.

Season generously and bring to a simmer. Simmer slowly for 1 hr until thick and saucy and the mince is tender. Serve with pasta and parmesan.

Tamarind prawn curry

Things Needed

1tbsp vegetable oil

1 onion, chopped

1 red chilli, finely chopped

garlic cloves, crushed

1tbsp ginger

1tsp turmeric

1tsp cumin seeds

1tsp ground coriander

400g cherry tomatoes

1tbsp tamarind paste (see tip, below)

250g raw king prawns

250g cooked basmati rice

Handful of coriander leaves, to serve

Direction

STEP 1

Heat the oil in a frying pan over a medium heat and cook the onion for 5-8 mins until light golden. Stir in the chilli, garlic and ginger, and fry for another minute before adding the spices. Tip in the cherry tomatoes, swirl the can out with a splash of water and stir that into the pan as well.

STEP 2

Simmer for 5 mins until the tomatoes burst and the sauce thickens. Stir in the tamarind and prawns, and simmer for 2-3 mins until the prawns are cooked. Serve the curry on top of the rice, with the coriander scattered over.

Smoky chickpeas on toast

Things Needed

1 tsp olive oil or vegetable oil, plus a drizzle

1 small onion or banana shallot, chopped

2 tsp chipotle paste

250ml passata

400g can chickpeas, drained

2 tsp honey

2 tsp red wine vinegar

2-4 slices good crusty bread

2 eggs

Direction

STEP 1

Heat ½ tsp of the oil in a pan. Tip in the onion and cook until soft, about 5-8 mins, then add the chipotle paste, passata, chickpeas, honey and vinegar. Season and bubble for 5 mins.

STEP 2

Toast the bread. Heat the remaining oil in a frying pan and fry the eggs. Drizzle the toast with a little oil, then top with the chickpeas and fried eggs.

Herby broccoli & pea soup

Things Needed

1 tbsp rapeseed oil

1 onion, finely chopped

1 large garlic clove, crushed

400g broccoli, chopped into small florets

300g frozen peas

200g chard, chopped

1l low-salt veg stock

½ small bunch of basil, chopped

small bunch of dill, chopped

1 lemon, zested and juiced

2 tbsp pumpkin seeds, toasted

Direction

STEP 1

Heat the oil in a large saucepan. Add the onion and fry for 8 mins until soft and translucent. Add the garlic and cook for 1 min more. Tip in the broccoli, peas and chard, then pour over the stock and bring the mixture to the boil. Reduce the heat to a simmer, cover and cook for 25 mins.

STEP 2

Stir through the herbs, lemon zest and juice, then blitz the soup with a stick blender until completely smooth. Ladle into bowls and serve with the toasted pumpkin seeds scattered over the top.

Tomato, pepper & bean one pot

Things Needed

1 tbsp olive oil

1 large onion, finely chopped

2 celery sticks, finely chopped

3 carrots, finely chopped

3 red peppers, sliced

2 garlic cloves, crushed

2 tbsp tomato purée

400g can cannellini beans, rinsed and drained

400g pinto beans, rinsed and drained

400g borlotti beans, rinsed and drained

2 x 400g cans chopped tomatoes

1 vegetable stock cube (check the label if you're vegan)

2 bay leaves

1 tbsp brown sugar

½ tbsp red wine vinegar

Direction

STEP 1

Heat the oil in a large pan or casserole on a medium heat. Fry the onion, celery and carrots for 10 mins until soft and golden, then add the peppers and fry for another 5 mins.

STEP 2

Stir in the garlic for a minute, then add the tomato purée, all the beans and chopped tomatoes, then swirl out the tomato cans with a splash of water and add to the pan with the stock cube, bay leaves, sugar and vinegar. Season and simmer, uncovered, for 25 mins until the sauce reduces to coat the beans and the peppers are soft. Leave to cool before storing in transportable containers. Will keep in the fridge for 3 - 4 days or freeze in portions and defrost in the fridge overnight.

Choose your toppings

Sweet & spicy

Add diced dried apricots and 1 tbsp harissa. Top with yogurt swirled with more harissa, and toasted flaked almonds.

Tex-Mex

Stir in ½ - 1 tbsp chipotle paste, shredded leftover roast chicken if you have any, and top with diced avocado, grated cheddar and coriander.

Smoky BBQ beans

Stir in 1 tbsp smoky BBQ sauce and crumble over shop-bought crispy bacon, a dollop of soured cream or yogurt, and some chopped herbs.

Added greens

Stir in some spinach and top with a sliced boiled egg.

Beans on toast

Serve the beans on toast or bread, add a dash of Tabasco or chilli flakes, crumble over feta and drizzle with olive oil.

Italian-inspired

Top with toasted croutons, chopped rosemary, lemon zest and parmesan

Pomegranate chicken with almond couscous

Things Needed

1 tbsp vegetable oil

200g couscous

1 chicken stock cube

1 large red onion, halved and thinly sliced

600g chicken mini fillets

4 tbsp tagine spice paste or 2 tbsp harissa

190ml bottle pomegranate juice (not sweetened; we used Pom Wonderful)

100g pack pomegranate seeds

100g pack toasted flaked almond

small pack mint, chopped

Direction

STEP 1

Boil the kettle and heat the oil in a large frying pan. Put the couscous in a bowl with some seasoning and crumble in half the stock cube. Add the onion to the pan and fry for a few mins to soften. Pour boiling water over the couscous to just cover, then cover the bowl with a tea towel and set aside.

STEP 2

Push the onion to one side of the pan, add the chicken fillets and brown on all sides. Stir in the tagine paste or harissa and the pomegranate juice, then crumble in the rest of the stock cube and season well. Simmer, uncovered, for 10 mins until the sauce has thickened and the chicken is cooked through. Stir through the pomegranate seeds, saving a few to scatter over before serving.

STEP 3

After 5 mins, fluff up the couscous with a fork and stir through the almonds and mint. Serve the chicken on the couscous with the sauce spooned over.

Air fryer halloumi

Things Needed

225g halloumi, cut into 6cm x 1cm thick slices

1 tsp olive oil

1 tsp smoked paprika, mixed herbs, or other flavourings (optional)

Our Most Popular Alternative

15-minute chicken & halloumi burgers

Direction

STEP 1

Heat your air fryer on 200C for 2 mins. Carefully pat the halloumi dry using kitchen paper or a clean cloth, then brush or rub with oil. Season with salt and pepper and any flavourings, if using.

STEP 2

Put the halloumi in the air fryer basket and cook for 8 mins until beginning to brown. Flip over and cook for a further 2-5 mins until crisp and golden.

Stir-fried chicken with broccoli & brown rice

Things Needed

200g trimmed broccoli florets (about 6), halved

1 chicken breast (approx 180g), diced

15g ginger, cut into shreds

2 garlic cloves, cut into shreds

1 red onion, sliced

1 roasted red pepper, from a jar, cut into cubes

2 tsp olive oil

1 tsp mild chilli powder

1 tbsp reduced-salt soy sauce

1 tbsp honey

250g pack cooked brown rice

Direction

STEP 1

Put the kettle on to boil and tip the broccoli into a medium pan ready to go on the heat. Pour the water over the broccoli then boil for 4 mins.

STEP 2

Heat the olive oil in a non-stick wok and stir-fry the ginger, garlic and onion for 2 mins, add the mild chilli powder and stir briefly. Add the chicken and stir-fry for 2 mins more. Drain the broccoli and reserve the water. Tip the broccoli into the wok with the soy, honey, red pepper and 4 tbsp broccoli water then cook until heated through. Meanwhile, heat the rice following the pack instructions and serve with the stir-fry.

MAIN DISH RECIPES ON STILLMAN DIET

Easy Spanish chicken

Things Needed

2 tbsp extra virgin olive oil

1 onion, thinly sliced

150g chorizo, cut into rings

1 red pepper, deseeded and sliced into strips

1 yellow pepper, deseeded and sliced into strips

1 tsp sweet smoked paprika

4 garlic cloves, finely chopped

400g can chopped tomatoes

150g pitted green olives

400g can butter beans, drained and rinsed

8 bone-in, skin-on chicken thighs

small handful of flat-leaf parsley, chopped

Direction

STEP 1

Heat the oven to 200C/180C fan/gas 6. Heat the olive oil in a large ovenproof frying pan over a medium heat and fry the onion, chorizo and peppers along with a pinch of salt and pepper for 15 mins until the veg has softened and the chorizo has released its oils. Add the paprika and garlic, and cook for another few minutes until fragrant.

STEP 2

Tip in the chopped tomatoes, olives and butter beans, stir to combine and season. Nestle in the chicken thighs and season well. Transfer to the oven and bake for 40 mins until the chicken skin is crisp and the meat cooked through and tender. Scatter with the parsley and serve.

Chicken chop suey

Things Needed

2 tbsp vegetable oil

1 large chicken breast, cut into thin bite-sized slices

1 onion, sliced

2 garlic cloves, roughly chopped or minced

1 carrot, sliced

½ tbsp dark soy sauce

½ tsp chicken powder or a pinch of salt

½ tsp sugar

pinch of white pepper (essential as it totally changes the flavour of the dish)

2 spring onions, chopped into slivers

100g ready-to-eat beansprouts

1 tbsp cornflour, mixed with 2 tbsp water

1 tsp sesame oil

steamed white rice or fried noodles, to serve

Direction

STEP 1

Heat a wok over a high heat and, once hot, pour in the oil. Add the chicken and fan out in a single layer so that it's in direct contact with the hot wok. Once it has started to brown on one side, give it a good stir, then toss in the onion and garlic. Stir, then add the carrots, dark soy, chicken powder or salt, sugar, white pepper and spring onions. Stir, then add the beansprouts and fry, stirring, for 1 min before pouring in 50ml just-boiled water.

STEP 2

Bring to the boil, then slowly pour in the cornflour paste to loosen it, mixing at the same time to prevent any lumps. Once the sauce has thickened, switch off the heat and add the sesame oil. Serve on a bed of steamed white rice or freshly fried noodles.

Fragrant lemongrass & coconut chicken stir-fry

Things Needed

1 lemongrass stick, outer husk removed, finely chopped (see tip, below)

15g ginger, peeled and grated

2 garlic cloves, crushed

1 lime, juiced

2 tsp light brown soft sugar

2 tbsp reduced-salt light soy sauce

60ml coconut water (or use water)

1 bird's-eye chilli, finely chopped (optional)

1 tbsp rapeseed oil

1 courgette, chopped

2 chicken breasts, thinly sliced

200g sugar snap peas, trimmed

15g desiccated coconut

250g pouch microwave wholegrain rice

Direction

STEP 1

Combine the lemongrass, ginger, garlic, lime juice, sugar, soy sauce, coconut water and chilli, if using, and set aside. Heat the oil in a wok

or large, high-sided pan over a high heat and stir-fry the courgette and chicken for 4 mins until browned. Stir in the peas and coconut and cook for 1-2 mins, stirring well to ensure the coconut doesn't burn.

STEP 2

Pour the lemongrass mixture around the edge of the pan, then stir in to combine. Continue to cook over a high heat for about 1-2 mins, until the chicken is cooked through and the sauce has reduced. Season to taste. Warm the rice following pack instructions, then serve with the stir-fry.

Air fryer steak

Things Needed

2 rib-eye steaks, around 260g each and 3cm thick

1 tsp oil

Our Most Popular Alternative

Air fryer crispy chilli beef

Direction

STEP 1

Dry off the steaks using kitchen paper or a clean cloth. Brush with the oil, then season generously with salt and freshly ground black pepper.

STEP 2

Heat the air fryer for 2 mins on 200C. Put the steaks in the basket and cook for 6 mins. Turn the steak and cook for a further 2 mins. At this point, your steak should be rare to medium rare. Cook for a further 2 mins for medium steaks, plus 2 mins more if you prefer them well-done.

STEP 3

Remove the steaks and put on a plate to rest for 3-4 mins. This is a perfect opportunity to make a sauce, if you like

Turmeric chicken with butter bean hummus & roasted peppers

Things Needed

1 large red pepper, halved and deseeded

1 tsp vegetable oil

160g long-stem broccoli

handful of mint leaves, to serve

For the chicken and marinade

2 large skinless chicken breast fillets (about 125g each)

120g natural yogurt

3 tbsp finely grated turmeric

½ tsp cumin seeds

½ tsp ground coriander

1 garlic clove, finely grated

1 tbsp lemon juice

1 tsp honey

1 tsp extra virgin olive oil

For the butter bean hummus

400g can butter beans, drained, liquid reserved

1 tbsp lemon zest, plus 1 tbsp lemon juice

1 tbsp extra virgin olive oil, plus a drizzle

1 garlic clove, roughly chopped

½ tsp cumin seeds

½ tsp ground coriander

Direction

STEP 1

Heat the oven to 220C/200C fan/gas 7. Line a baking sheet with foil. Make a few small cuts around the edges of the pepper halves using a sharp knife, then flatten them as much as you can with your palm. Rub with the veg oil and roast on the lined baking sheet for 10 mins.

STEP 2

Meanwhile, cut the chicken breasts in half lengthways at an angle so you end up with four thin fillets. Mix the yogurt, turmeric, cumin seeds, ground coriander, garlic, lemon juice, honey and olive oil with some black pepper and 1 tsp salt in a bowl. Add the chicken and turn to coat in the marinade. When the peppers have had 10 mins, turn them over, add the chicken fillets to the sheet, spacing them apart slightly, and spoon any remaining marinade over them. Roast for 20 mins, turning the chicken fillets halfway, until cooked through.

STEP 3

For the hummus, use a hand blender to blitz together the beans, lemon zest and juice, olive oil, garlic, cumin seeds and coriander with 6 tbsp liquid from the can, ¾ tsp salt and plenty of black pepper. It should be completely smooth.

STEP 4

When the chicken has been cooking for 10 mins, steam the broccoli for 6 mins until tender. Spoon the hummus over two plates, then top with the roasted peppers and chicken.

Scatter with the mint, drizzle with olive oil and serve with the broccoli on the side.

One-pot cheeseburger pasta

Things Needed

1 tbsp olive oil

1 large onion, chopped

500g minced beef

2 tomatoes, chopped

1 tbsp Worcestershire sauce

500ml warm beef stock

300g fusilli or other pasta shape

100ml milk

125g mature cheddar, coarsely grated, plus extra to serve

1 tbsp mustard

1 tbsp ketchup, plus extra to serve

50-70g pickles, chopped

sliced dill pickles and/or jalapeños, to serve

Direction

STEP 1

Heat the oil in a large lidded saucepan over a medium heat. Fry the onion for 3 mins, then add the mince and cook for a further 5 mins until lightly browned.

STEP 2

Add the tomatoes and Worcestershire sauce and cook for 2 mins until the tomatoes are pulpy and starting to soften. Pour in the stock and bring to the boil.

STEP 3

Stir in the pasta, then cover and cook for 10-12 mins until the pasta is tender and the liquid has mostly been absorbed, adding a splash of water if needed.

STEP 4

Pour in the milk and stir in 100g of the cheese, stirring until melted. Check the seasoning and transfer to a serving dish or bowls. Drizzle with mustard and ketchup, then scatter with the remaining cheese, pickles and jalapeños and a good grinding of black pepper. Serve with more ketchup on the side.

Cabbage rolls

Things Needed

1 white cabbage

300g rice

1 large onion, finely chopped

2 tbsp olive oil

750g pork mince

1 egg

pinch of dried marjoram

200g tomato purée

Direction

STEP 1

Bring a pan of salted water to the boil. Cut the base off the cabbage and cook it whole in the boiling water for about 4 mins. Remove the outer leaves, then keep peeling away more and set them aside. You may need to cook the heart of the cabbage a little longer to un-peel the innermost leaves. Or if you prefer, cut the leaves off the raw cabbage and cook them loose for 1-2 mins. Reserve the cooking water.

STEP 2

Cook the rice according to pack instruction and drain it well – it needs to be very dry. Fry the onion in the oil for 8 -10 mins or until soft and cooked through. Put the pork, rice, onions egg and marjoram in a bowl, season well and mix thoroughly.

STEP 3

Lay out each cabbage leaf and put 2 heaped tbsp of stuffing in the centre towards the stalk end. Fold in the sides, then roll up tightly. Repeat with the remaining mixture and leaves.

STEP 4

Cover the base of a deep, wide pan with the smaller cabbage leaves. Pack the cabbage rolls on top of the leaves, tightly together. Then, make a tomato sauce by mixing the tomato purée with some salt and pepper and some of the reserved cabbage water. You need enough to submerge the cabbage rolls by a couple of centimetres. Simmer, covered, for 2 hrs. Serve the cabbage rolls with the tomato sauce.

Sloppy joes

Things Needed

1tbsp vegetable oil

1 onion, finely chopped

2 small red peppers or yellow peppers, finely chopped

400g minced beef

2 x 400g cans chopped tomatoes

4tbsp Nando's PERi-BBQ sauce

4 cheese slices

6 burger buns

crispy onions, to serve

tbsp iceberg lettuce, to serve

Direction

STEP 1

Heat the oil in a deep frying pan, and tip in the mince, breaking it up with a wooden spoon as you go, until browned all over. Stir in the onion and pepper and cook for 8-10 mins until softened. Tip in the tomatoes and Nando's PERi-BBQ sauce, and season. Simmer for 20-25 mins until the sauce has thickened.

STEP 2

Put the cheese slices on top of the mince and cover with a lid for 2 mins to let it melt into the sauce. Pile into the buns with the crispy onions, and lettuce on the side for scooping up the extra sauce.

Chorizo & chickpea summer stew

Things Needed

1 tbsp olive oil

2 garlic cloves, crushed

2 thyme sprigs

1 tbsp smoked paprika

200g chorizo ring, sliced into thin coins

1 tbsp sherry vinegar

600g cherry tomatoes, halved

450g jar roasted red peppers, drained and cut
into large strips

100g spinach

2 x 400g cans chickpeas, drained

drizzle of extra virgin olive oil and crusty bread, to serve

Direction

STEP 1

Heat the oil in a large frying pan over a medium heat, add the garlic, thyme and smoked paprika, and stir for a few minutes, then tip in the chorizo and stir for another couple of minutes until its oil is released. Splash in the sherry vinegar and let it bubble for a minute or so.

STEP 2

Add the tomatoes, peppers, spinach and chickpeas along with 100ml water and a pinch of seasoning. Bring to the boil, then reduce the heat to a simmer and cook until the tomatoes have softened and there is a thickened sauce, about 15 mins. Adjust the seasoning and finish with a drizzle of extra virgin olive oil. Serve with crusty bread

Chicken nuggets

Things Needed

400g chicken breast fillets

4 tbsp plain flour

1 egg, lightly beaten

115g panko breadcrumbs or other dried breadcrumbs

2 tbsp vegetable or sunflower oil

Direction

STEP 1

Cut the chicken into bite-sized pieces and place the pieces between two layers of baking paper. Use a rolling pin to gently flatten the pieces until they are around 2-3mm thick and uniform.

STEP 2

Tip the flour onto a plate and mix it with a pinch of salt. Put the beaten egg in a bowl, and tip the breadcrumbs into another bowl. For the air fryer Direction, lightly oil a large baking tray.

STEP 3

Dip each chicken piece in the flour, then into the egg (shaking off the excess), and finally toss in the breadcrumbs. Transfer the coated chicken pieces to a lightly oiled baking tray for the oven Direction or the air fryer basket for the air fryer Direction. Breadcrumbing using one hand is less messy.

STEP 4

If you're using the oven, not pan-frying, preheat it to 220C/200C fan/gas 7. Bake the nuggets for 10-15 mins, turning them halfway through.

STEP 5

If you're using the air-fryer, preheat it to 200C for 4 mins. Brush the chicken pieces on both sides with oil. Cook the nuggets in batches in the air-fryer basket for 5 mins per batch until golden and crunchy. Shake the basket halfway through to ensure even cooking.

STEP 6

Serve the chicken nuggets with tomato sauce, if you like.

Chicken sausage pasta

Things Needed

1 tbsp sunflower oil

1 onion, chopped

400g chicken sausage, sliced

1 large garlic clove, crushed or finely grated

200g roasted red peppers, chopped

1 tsp ground cumin (optional)

½ tsp chilli flakes (optional)

400g can chopped tomatoes

100g spinach

500g penne or rigatoni pasta

Direction

STEP 1

Heat the oil in a large lidded frying pan or saucepan over a medium heat and fry the onion for 5 mins until beginning to soften. Tip in the sausage pieces and fry for 4-5 mins until beginning to brown. Tip in the garlic, peppers, cumin and chilli, if using, season well and stir to combine. Cook for 2-3 mins more until fragrant, then tip in the chopped tomatoes and half a can of water. Reduce the heat to a simmer and cook for another 10-15 mins until the liquid has reduced a little and the sausages are cooked through. Add the spinach, stir, cover and cook for 3-5 mins more until the spinach has wilted, then mix to combine.

STEP 2

Meanwhile, cook the pasta following pack instructions. Drain, reserving a cupful of the pasta water.

STEP 3

Tip the cooked pasta into the sauce and stir gently to combine. Cook for a 2-3 mins, then stir in some of the reserved pasta water if the sauce needs to be loosened. Serve.

Ukrainian pork rib borsch

Things Needed

1.5kg pork ribs

2 onions

1 medium beetroot, peeled and cut into matchsticks

2 tbsp vegetable oil (optional)

2 medium carrots, grated

4 medium potatoes, chopped

2 tbsp tomato purée

400g can chopped tomatoes

1 bay leaf

400g white cabbage, sliced

2 celery sticks, chopped

1 large red pepper, sliced

1 tbsp chopped parsley

2 garlic cloves, crushed (optional)

1 whole chilli (optional)

1 tbsp chopped dill

100ml soured cream or crème fraîche (optional)

crusty bread, to serve

Direction

STEP 1

Put the ribs in a large saucepan and pour over 3 litres cold water, then season with salt. Bring to the boil over a medium heat, skimming off any foam that rises to the surface. Peel one of the onions and add this to the pan whole, along with the beetroot. Reduce the heat to low and simmer for 1 hr-1 hr 15 mins until the meat is tender. If the ribs don't have much fat, they will need to cook for longer. Remove the whole onion and compost it.

STEP 2

Meanwhile, make zasmażka – a Ukrainian sofrito. Skim 2 tbsp fat off the ribs as they cook, and pour it into a large frying pan (or use 2 tbsp vegetable oil). Finely chop the second onion and fry it over a low-medium heat, stirring often for about 5 mins until transparent and soft. Add the grated carrots and cook for 10 mins more. Tip in the potatoes and stir in the tomato purée. Pour in the canned tomatoes and cook for 5 mins, then taste and add 1-2 tsp sugar to balance out the acidity, if needed. Add the bay leaf.

STEP 3

When the potato is soft (don't worry if it overcooks, it will give body to the borsch), add the zasmażka to the ribs and stock, and bring to the boil again. Add the cabbage, celery, pepper and parsley, and cook for 7 mins – try not to overcook the cabbage.

STEP 4

Mash the garlic, if using, with a pinch of salt to make a paste, then add this to the borsch for more flavour. Stir in the whole chilli, if using, and continue to cook briefly to warm through slightly.

STEP 5

Shred the meat using two forks and remove and discard the bones. Serve the borsch in bowls, each topped with 1 tbsp of the soured cream and some chopped dill, with some crusty bread on the side, if you like.

Chicken & pasta bake

Things Needed

2 tbsp olive oil

100g smoked streaky bacon, cut into small pieces

4 chicken breasts, cut into chunks

1 red onion, finely chopped

2 garlic cloves, finely chopped

1 red pepper, diced

1 yellow pepper, diced

1 tsp oregano

¼ tsp chilli flakes (optional)

2 x 400g cans chopped tomatoes

1 tsp caster sugar

small bunch of parsley, roughly chopped

3 tbsp mascarpone

350g pasta, any shape – if long, snap them in half

65g cheddar, grated

50g mozzarella, grated

Direction

STEP 1

Heat the oil in a large, wide casserole, over a medium heat. Stir in the bacon and cook for 5-7 mins, until crispy and browned. Remove to a bowl using a slotted spoon and set aside. Tip in the chicken and stir well to coat in the bacon fat. Turn the heat up to medium-high and cook for 3-5 mins until browned all over (it doesn't need to be cooked through at this point). Remove to the same bowl as the bacon using a slotted spoon.

STEP 2

Mix the onion and garlic in with a pinch of salt and turn the heat down to medium. Cook for 10-12 mins until softened. Add the peppers, oregano and chilli flakes, if using. Cook for a further 8-10 mins until the peppers have softened. Pour in the canned tomatoes, then swill out the cans with a little water and tip this in as well. Sprinkle over the sugar and stir in the chicken and bacon and most of the parsley. Season well and bring to a simmer. Cook for

20-25 mins, until thickened. Mix in the mascarpone, stirring well until dissolved.

STEP 3

Meanwhile, cook the pasta for 2 mins less than the pack states, then drain thoroughly reserving a mug of the pasta cooking water. Heat the oven to 220C/200C fan/gas 7. Taste and season the sauce before tipping in the cooked pasta. Pour in a splash of the pasta cooking water to bring the sauce together before spooning the mixture into an ovenproof baking dish. Will keep covered and frozen for up to three months. Defrost thoroughly in the fridge overnight before baking. Top with both cheeses and bake for 10-15 mins until golden and bubbling. Scatter over the remaining parsley and serve straight from the dish.

Bigos (Polish hunter's stew)

Things Needed

1 white cabbage finely sliced

250ml beef stock

100g dried mushrooms, soaked in boiling water for 1 hr

2 tbsp lard

400g German-style sausages, sliced

250g smoked bacon, diced or sliced

2 onions, chopped

750g cooked pork, game meat or beef, diced

200g prunes

1 bay leaf

2 cloves

12 peppercorns

4 juniper berries

4 allspice berries

90ml red wine

2 tbsp tomato purée

Direction

STEP 1

Put the cabbage in a heavy casserole dish, add the stock and cook over a low heat for about 50 mins, until tender.

STEP 2

Cut the soaked mushrooms into strips and save the soaking water. Heat the lard and fry the sausages and bacon, then scoop out, leaving the fat in the pan. Fry the onion in the same pan for 5-8 mins until lightly browned.

STEP 3

Add the mushrooms and their liquid along with all the cooked meat, onions and prunes, then cover and cook for 20 mins. Add the spices, red wine and tomato purée and bring to a simmer, then cover and cook for 1 hr. Season well and leave to cool. Will keep covered and chilled for up to two days. Bigos improves in flavour over a couple of days. Leave to cool first. Reheat until piping hot before serving

Chicken tikka

Things Needed

3 large chicken breasts, cut into chunks

75g Greek yogurt

2 tbsp ginger and garlic paste

1 tbsp madras curry powder

1 tsp ground cumin

1 tsp ground coriander

1 tsp ground turmeric

1 tsp smoked paprika

2 tsp mild chilli powder

1 tbsp lemon juice

Direction

STEP 1

Tip all of the Things Needed into a large bowl with a big pinch of salt and pepper and mix well. Cover and chill for at least a few hours, but preferably overnight.

STEP 2

Heat the grill or a barbecue to high. Thread the chicken pieces onto four metal skewers, packing the pieces in so they're all touching. Put onto a baking tray under the grill, or onto the grills of the barbecue and cook for 4-5 mins, until charred, then flip and repeat.

SECTION 6: POTENTIAL HAZARDS AND CONSIDERATIONS

Prior to embarking on the Stillman Diet, it's imperative for individuals to thoroughly comprehend the potential risks and concerns associated with this particular weight loss regimen, as is prudent with any form of restrictive dietary approach. Assessing whether the Stillman Diet aligns with one's health goals and lifestyle necessitates a comprehensive understanding of its various components and implications.

A primary concern surrounding the Stillman Diet revolves around the risk of nutritional deficiencies. Given its emphasis on high protein intake and carbohydrate restriction, there's a possibility that individuals may consume insufficient quantities of fruits, vegetables, and whole grains — essential sources of fiber, vitamins, and minerals. Neglecting to maintain nutritional balance while strictly adhering to the diet over an extended period could precipitate deficiencies, potentially compromising overall health.

Additionally, there's apprehension regarding the potential strain placed on the kidneys due to the diet's elevated protein content. Individuals with pre-existing kidney issues or a familial history of kidney disease may face heightened risks, as a protein-rich diet may exacerbate renal problems. Consequently, it's advisable for such individuals to exercise caution and consult with a healthcare professional before embarking on a high-protein diet regimen.

The restrictive nature of the Stillman Diet may pose challenges to long-term adherence, potentially resulting in monotony in food choices and subsequent deviations from the prescribed eating plan. The lack of dietary variety could lead to boredom and temptation to stray from healthy eating habits, undermining weight loss efforts in the long run. Thus, it's essential to select dietary patterns that are sustainable over time to prevent potential boredom and ensure adherence to weight loss goals.

Moreover, the transition to a reduced carbohydrate intake and subsequent induction of ketosis may predispose individuals to dehydration, particularly during the initial stages of the diet. Adequate hydration is crucial to mitigate potential adverse effects such as headaches, lethargy, and constipation, underscoring the importance of maintaining proper fluid intake throughout the dietary regimen.

Individuals considering the Stillman Diet should be aware of these potential pitfalls, which encompass kidney health concerns, dietary monotony, and dehydration risks. Prioritizing personalized health evaluations and seeking individualized guidance from healthcare providers or certified dietitians is recommended before embarking on any restrictive dietary regimen. Furthermore, exploring sustainable and balanced nutritional alternatives may offer a more viable long-term approach for weight management endeavors.

Incorporating Physical Activities

Incorporating physical activity into your routine while following the Stillman Diet is not only crucial for overall health improvement but also enhances the efficacy of weight loss endeavors. While the diet primarily focuses on macronutrient composition, regular exercise complements its approach by contributing to a comprehensive and sustainable weight management strategy.

Weight loss necessitates creating a calorie deficit, and exercise plays a pivotal role in achieving this goal. Engaging in aerobic workouts, strength training, or a combination of both can elevate total energy expenditure, thereby facilitating the caloric deficit essential for shedding excess weight.

Furthermore, exercise aids in the preservation of lean muscle mass, particularly significant when protein intake is emphasized in the diet. Maintaining muscle mass is essential for a healthy metabolism, as muscles burn more calories even at rest compared to fat tissue. Strength training activities are particularly beneficial in this regard.

Beyond weight loss, regular physical activity also confers numerous health benefits, including improvements in cardiovascular health, endurance, mood, and sleep quality. These benefits complement the weight reduction focus of the Stillman Diet, contributing to an overall sense of well-being.

It's essential to consider timing and intensity of exercise, especially during the initial stages of the Stillman Diet when the body adjusts to lower carbohydrate intake and enters a state of ketosis. Adjusting the intensity and duration of physical activity may be necessary for individuals experiencing temporary fatigue during this transition.

Adding exercise to the Stillman Diet not only accelerates weight loss but also enhances overall well-being, promoting a healthier and more balanced lifestyle. It's crucial for individuals to engage in physical activities they enjoy and can sustain, gradually increasing intensity as their bodies adapt to the dietary changes.

To ensure that the exercise regimen aligns with individual needs and goals, seeking guidance from a healthcare provider or fitness specialist is advisable, particularly for those with pre-existing health conditions or concerns. Tailoring the exercise program to specific requirements enhances safety and efficacy, facilitating long-term adherence and maximizing health outcomes.

SECTION 7: ACHIEVING YOUR GOALS ON THE STILLMAN DIET

If you're seeking an innovative approach to weight loss, the Stillman Diet presents itself as a potential option, placing emphasis on protein consumption while restricting carbohydrates. However, before embarking on this dietary regimen, it is essential to carefully consider the potential hazards and challenges it may entail, notwithstanding its ability to yield rapid initial results.

Among the considerations to bear in mind are the risks of nutritional deficiencies, strain on renal health, dietary monotony, and the imperative need for adequate hydration. Despite its promise of swift weight reduction, transitioning off the Stillman Diet requires a gradual reintroduction of a diverse range of foods, all while maintaining a focus on healthy eating habits and portion control.

Throughout this dietary journey, it is crucial to incorporate physical activity as a fundamental component to promote overall health and sustain weight loss achievements. The high-protein, low-carbohydrate principles underlying the Stillman Diet can impact various aspects of health, including metabolism, appetite regulation, and muscle preservation.

Potential concerns such as nutritional imbalances and renal stress should be carefully deliberated in consultation with healthcare professionals. Furthermore, staying well-hydrated is paramount for optimal digestion, hunger regulation, and metabolic function, complementing the benefits of the Stillman Diet.

Incorporating regular exercise into the regimen not only aids in calorie expenditure but also helps in preserving lean muscle mass and enhancing cardiovascular health, synergistically reinforcing the dietary efforts.

Before embarking on or discontinuing the Stillman Diet, it is imperative to assess individual health status, preferences, and goals. A holistic and sustainable approach to weight management entails embracing a well-rounded lifestyle regimen encompassing balanced nutrition, adequate hydration, regular physical activity, and ongoing medical supervision.

By integrating these elements into a comprehensive plan tailored to individual needs, one can strive towards achieving and maintaining a healthy weight in the long term, prioritizing both physical and mental well-being.

Moving away from the Stillman Diet

Transitioning away from the Stillman Diet to embrace a healthier and more diverse dietary pattern requires thoughtful consideration and planning to minimize any potential discomfort. The rigid guidelines of the Stillman Diet, characterized by low carbohydrate intake and an emphasis on high protein consumption, can pose challenges without careful preparation.

A crucial aspect of this transition involves gradually reintroducing a broader spectrum of foods into one's diet. After initially restricting protein-heavy meals, individuals can gradually incorporate nutrient-rich options such as fruits, vegetables, and whole grains. This gradual reintroduction helps address any potential nutrient deficiencies that may have arisen during the adherence to the Stillman Diet, particularly in terms of fiber, vitamins, and minerals.

Furthermore, it's essential to monitor macronutrient ratios during this transition period. Instead of abruptly increasing carbohydrate intake, a gradual approach that ensures adequate intake of fats and proteins is recommended. This gradual adjustment allows the body to adapt more smoothly to changes in dietary composition.

Portion control remains paramount throughout this transition. While expanding food choices, it's crucial to monitor portion sizes to prevent overconsumption. By practicing portion control, individuals can foster a sustainable and balanced eating routine that supports long-term weight management goals.

Seeking guidance from healthcare professionals or certified dietitians is advisable during this transition phase. These experts can provide personalized recommendations tailored to individual health conditions, dietary preferences, and weight loss objectives. By avoiding extreme dieting measures, individuals can receive guidance on maintaining weight loss while ensuring adequate nutrient intake for overall health and well-being.

In addition to dietary adjustments, establishing a consistent pattern of physical exercise is essential. Regular physical activity not only supports weight management but also offers numerous health benefits. Choosing enjoyable activities that align with personal preferences can help maintain a lifelong commitment to physical fitness as part of a healthy lifestyle.

In conclusion, transitioning away from the Stillman Diet involves a gradual reintroduction of diverse foods, careful monitoring of macronutrient ratios, portion control, consultation with healthcare professionals, and incorporation of regular physical activity. By adopting a balanced and sustainable approach to eating and exercise, individuals can achieve long-term health and weight management beyond the confines of restrictive dietary patterns.

SECTION 8: IN SUMMARY!

The Stillman Diet represents a notable dietary approach that has garnered attention for its focus on high-protein, low-carbohydrate consumption to stimulate rapid weight loss. Throughout our exploration of this regimen, we've observed its potential benefits and considerations, shedding light on both its strengths and limitations.

While the Stillman Diet demonstrates efficacy in initiating rapid weight loss, its sustainability and long-term feasibility warrant careful examination. The restrictive nature of the diet, primarily centered around protein-rich foods while severely limiting carbohydrates and fats, may pose challenges in maintaining adherence over extended periods. Furthermore, concerns regarding potential nutritional deficiencies, particularly in essential vitamins, minerals, and dietary fiber, underscore the importance of close monitoring and supplementation where necessary.

Beyond its nutritional implications, the Stillman Diet also raises questions about its compatibility with individual lifestyles, preferences, and medical considerations. Potential side effects such as fatigue, constipation, and muscle loss, coupled with the risk of metabolic imbalances, highlight the need for personalized guidance and oversight when embarking on this dietary regimen.

Nevertheless, the Stillman Diet offers a structured framework that may appeal to individuals seeking rapid weight loss or those motivated by quick results. Its emphasis on protein intake can provide a sense of satiety and may support muscle preservation during periods of calorie restriction. However, it is essential to approach this approach with caution and to consider its potential risks and benefits within the context of overall health and well-being.

In light of these considerations, individuals contemplating the Stillman Diet are encouraged to consult with healthcare professionals or registered dietitians to assess its appropriateness for their unique needs and circumstances. Furthermore, incorporating principles of balanced nutrition, regular physical activity, and mindful eating habits remains fundamental to achieving sustainable weight management outcomes in the long term.

Ultimately, while the Stillman Diet may serve as a temporary tool for initiating weight loss, it is essential to prioritize holistic health and wellness, embracing approaches that promote both physical and emotional well-being for lasting success on the journey toward optimal health.

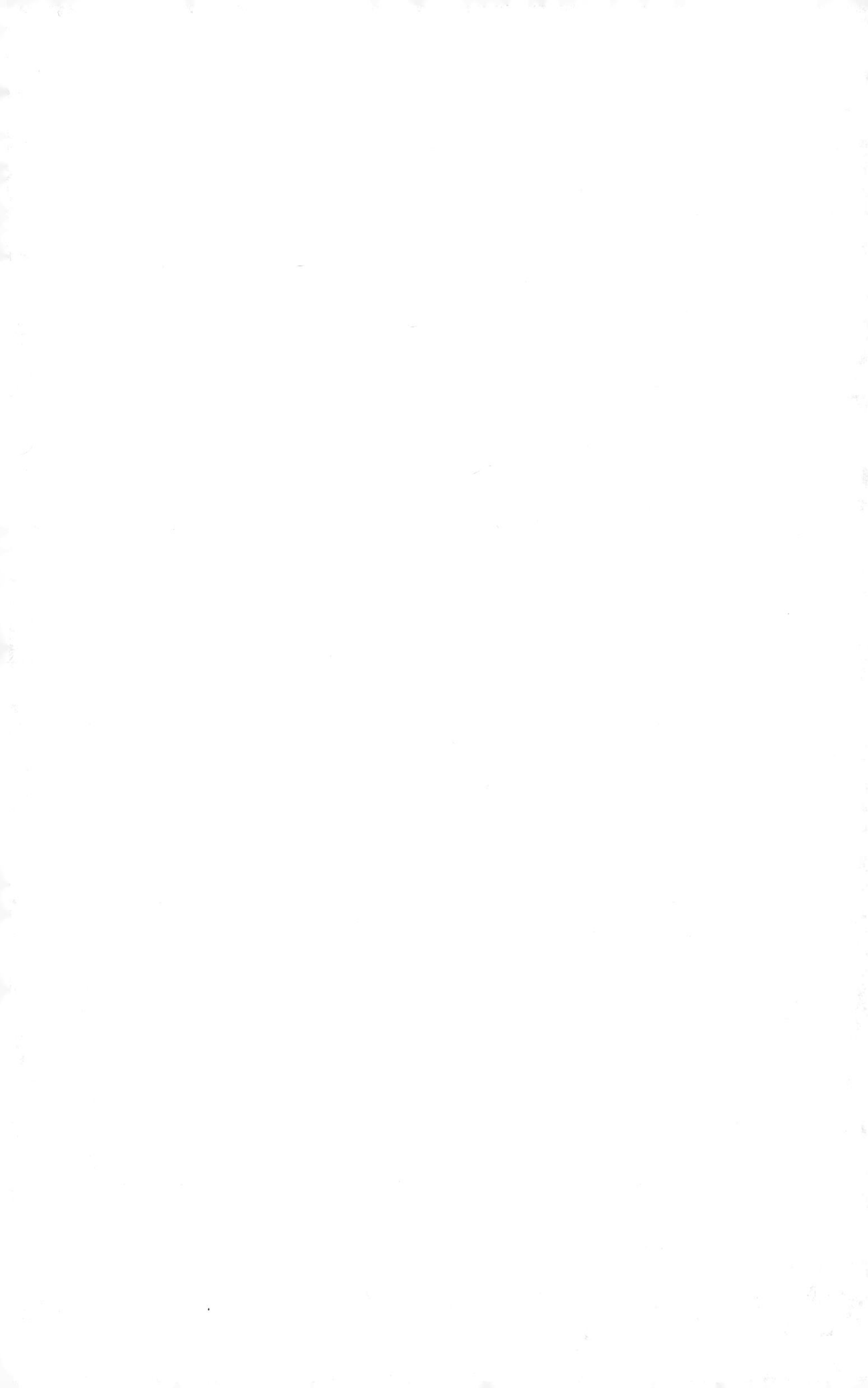